Middlesex Memories

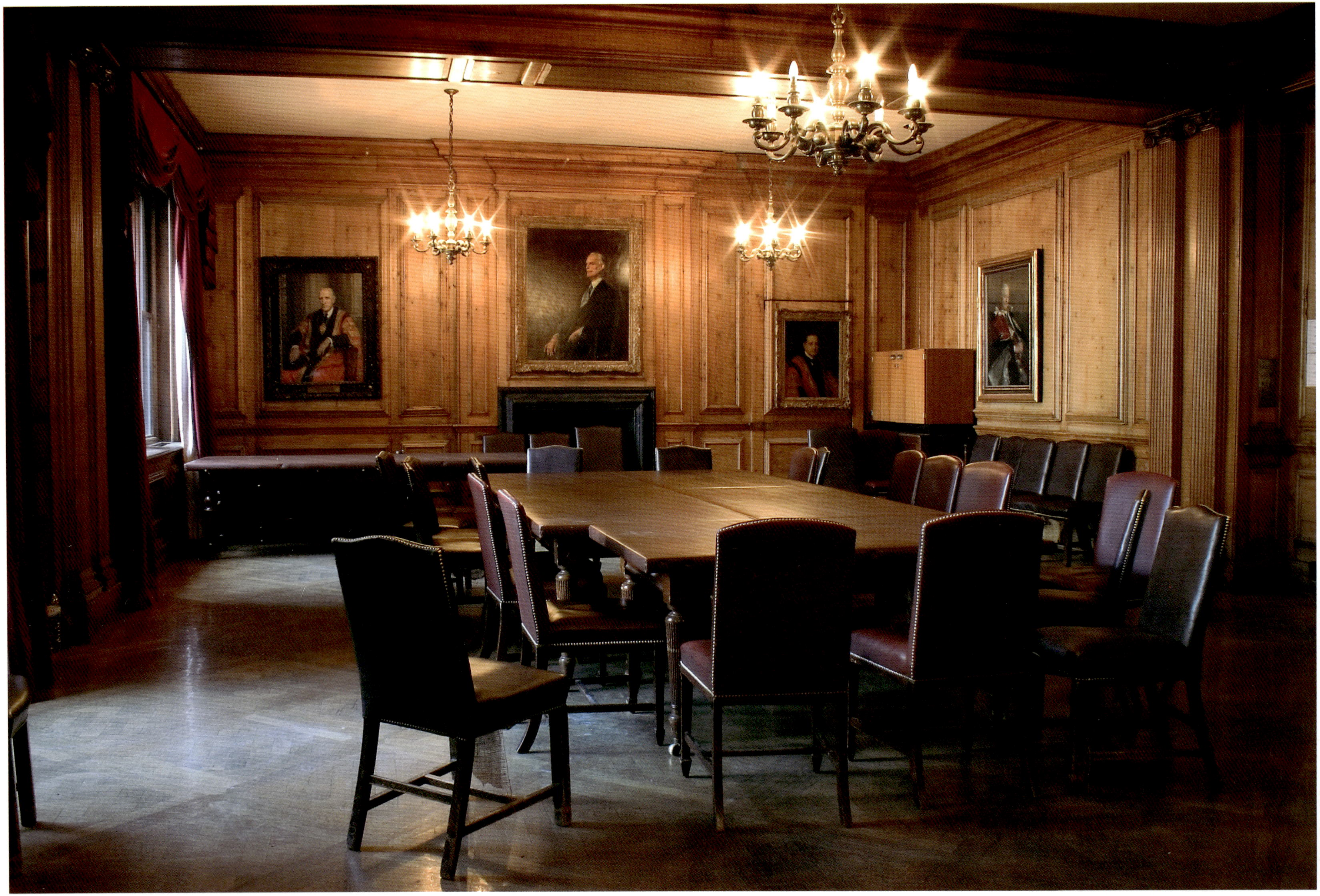

Middlesex Memories

Carole Rawlinson

University College London Hospitals Charities

Carole Rawlinson's photographic work has developed in parallel with a long career as a hospital planner. An Associate of the Royal Photographic Association, she is a member of Hampstead Photographic Society and London Independent Photography and her work has been shown in several exhibitions. Carole is a stock photographer for the Royal Geographical Society Picture Library which holds a wide selection of her wild places images. Her interest in The Middlesex Hospital has been both professional and personal. She was a member of Bloomsbury Health Authority in the late 80s and her daughters were both born in The Middlesex.

First published in 2007 by University College London Hospitals Charities

www.carolerawlinson.co.uk

ISBN 978-0-9555689-0-9

Designer Robert Updegraff
Production Management Geoff Barlow
Origination XY Digital Limited
Printed in Hong Kong

Contents

Acknowledgements

I am very grateful to many individuals – past and present staff, members of the former Board and Health Authority and patients who spent time sharing their memories of The Middlesex with me. I am also indebted to Peter Burroughs, then Capital Development Director, UCLH and Louise Boden, Chief Nurse, UCLH and their colleagues, for facilitating my access to The Middlesex during the hospital closure process in 2005. Thanks are also due to Guy Noble, Arts Curator, UCLH Arts for sponsoring this book and the associated exhibition and to University College London Hospital Charities for funding the publication of this book. Finally, I would like to thank Annie Lindsay, UCLH archivist for background information on The Middlesex and advice on the history summary and Peter Dixon, Chair, University College London Hospitals NHS Foundation Trust for writing the Foreword to this book.

Carole Rawlinson *June 2007*

Foreword

When I first saw the photograph of the old Middlesex Hospital clock which was used as the invitation to Carole Rawlinson's photographic exhibition I knew we were on to something special. When I went to the opening of the exhibition itself in the Street Gallery in the new UCH I knew at once that we should find a way of making a permanent record of a wonderful series of images that capture the life and the importance of The Middlesex.

This book is the result. Thanks to funding from our charitable trustees and Carole's generosity, we have been able to publish this collection for a wider audience and I am delighted to contribute this foreword.

Given the many distinguished men and women who have been part of the history of The Middlesex I feel particularly poorly qualified but I do at least have an appreciation of its importance and my own warm memories. I well remember chairing board meetings under the steely gaze of Lord Astor's portrait, a daunting prospect. I remember my first visit to the tunnels and wondering if I would ever find my way out. The painted yellow line never seemed much help to me. I remember the midnight service at Christmas in the glorious chapel with my family and a few staff and patients, often very obviously unwell. Others will have their own memories and I am quite sure that the pictures in this book will bring them flooding back.

Those who take the view that history is bunk are missing a trick. History is the DNA of the present and while the old hospital may be closed, the legacy of The Middlesex lives on and its wonderful record of service over 250 years is commemorated, not just in the name of the tower in the new building on Euston Road, but in so many other ways, including now this splendid volume.

My thanks and congratulations to everyone who has had a role in producing it.

Peter Dixon, *Chairman, University College London Hospitals NHS Foundation Trust*

Introduction

This book provides a snapshot in time of this well loved teaching hospital as it went out of use as a major healthcare facility at the end of 2005. The history of The Middlesex stretches back over 250 years but this famous building has finally been left behind by modern healthcare developments.

The book links images of parts of The Middlesex Hospital building to people's memories of the hospital at particular points in their lives as staff or patients.

The aim of the book is to evoke personal memories of The Middlesex on the part of readers, rather than to provide a comprehensive historical record.

The photographs were taken between August and November 2005 as The Middlesex was vacated by patients but still retained its healthcare characteristics.

Carole Rawlinson *June 2007*

The Middlesex Hospital 1745 – 2006

History Headlines

1745 Foundation of the Middlesex Infirmary which opened on Windmill Street with 18 beds

1746 The Middlesex Infirmary was renamed The Middlesex Hospital, one of 5 voluntary general hospitals in London, and inpatient capacity was increased to 40 beds

1755 Foundation stone laid for a new Middlesex hospital with 64 beds which opened on Mortimer Street in 1757. East and West wings opened in 1766 and 1780

1774 The Medical Society was formed by Middlesex students, the second oldest medical society in the UK

1828 Links between The Middlesex and University College were rejected

1834 North London Hospital opened and was renamed University College Hospital in 1837

1835 The Middlesex Hospital Medical School was founded

1844 The Hospital for Diseases of Women opened and was renamed The Hospital for Women in 1845

1854 The Middlesex dealt with a major cholera outbreak around Soho

1856 Dr Temple Frere was appointed the first Dean of The Middlesex Hospital Medical School

1860 Elizabeth Garret Anderson began part of her medical training at The Middlesex

1870 Miss Godiva Thorold was appointed matron and introduced traditions, standards of excellence and uniforms for nursing at The Middlesex

1889 The new Hospital for Women moved to a new building on Euston Road

1890 The Middlesex Chapel was built

1896 The Middlesex Hospital amalgamated with its Medical School

1901 The first X-ray machine was acquired by The Middlesex

1905 The new UCH building, known as the Cruciform, was completed on Gower Street

1912 The Ladies Work Society was established at The Middlesex. This became The Ladies Association in 1921 and the League of Friends in 1968

1914 Sir John Bland Sutton funded the building of the Institute of Pathology. Many staff served in the forces during World War I

1917 The new Hospital for Women was renamed the Elizabeth Garret Anderson Hospital

1920 Frederick Cayley Robinson completed the Acts of Mercy paintings which were transferred to the new Middlesex hospital and hung in main reception when it was opened in 1935

1924 The Middlesex Hospital buildings were declared unsafe – the 'Falling Down' notice was issued and a rebuild appeal launched

1926 The Poor Law Infirmary, already acquired on Cleveland Street, was used for inpatients and outpatients during rebuilding of The Middlesex

1927 The Ferens Institute of Otolaryngology opened on the top floor of the Outpatients Department

1928 The Courtauld Institute of Biochemistry opened

1931 Lord Astor funded a new nurses' home built off The Middlesex island site (named John Astor House in 1948)

1934 The Middlesex Hospital rebuilding appeal was ended dramatically by Sir Edward Myerstein who donated the outstanding appeal sum

1934 Sister Dorothy Thomas received the Empire Gallantry Medal, later upgraded to George Cross, for extinguishing a blazing oxygen cylinder in a Middlesex anaesthetic room

1935 The new Middlesex Hospital, costing £1.25m, re-opened on present site with 715 beds, its East wing devoted to medical cases and the West wing to surgical cases. Research and education facilities were provided in the crosspiece

1940 The top 3 floors of The Middlesex Hospital were closed during the blitz. Many staff served in the forces during World War II

1946 Brigadier Hardy Roberts was appointed as Secretary Superintendent and Miss Marjorie Marriot as Matron

1948 Following the formation of the NHS, management of The Middlesex Medical School and Hospital became separated. The Middlesex Hospital Group of Teaching Hospital was established and formal associations made with St Luke's Woodside, The Hospital for Women and the British Red Cross Society's Clinic for Rheumatism (Arthur Stanley Institute)

1958 Athlone House, a Middlesex recovery unit, opened in Highgate

1959 The Macdonald-Buchanan School of Nursing was built and the first phase of the Windeyer building to house The Middlesex Medical School

1965 James Pringle House and Arthur Stanley House opened

1974 NHS reorganisation. The Board of Governors were abolished and new regional, area and district health authorities established. Sir Jules Thorne Institute of Clinical Science built on the Middlesex island site

1979 The Wolfson Building was completed for Middlesex School and Hospital Psychiatry departments

1982 NHS reorganisation put both The Middlesex and University College Hospital into the new Bloomsbury Health Authority. Agreement in principle reached to form a Joint Medical School. Casualty department closed and service moved to UCH. Hospital for Women beds transferred to The Elizabeth Garrett Anderson Hospital. All obstetric services were transferred from the Middlesex to UCH

1983 The 25 Club was formed

1984 Final agreement was reached to form a single School of Medicine within UCL. This opened in 1987

1986 The Middlesex and University College Schools of Nursing became the Bloomsbury and Islington College of Nursing and Midwifery

1989 The Hospital for Women, Soho Square closed and its services were amalgamated with the Elizabeth Garret Anderson Hospital

1992 The St Peter's Group of hospitals was closed and services moved to The Middlesex

1994 The Middlesex Hospital became part of the new UCL Hospitals NHS Trust which also included the EGA and the Hospital for Tropical Diseases. UCH Cruciform building was closed and was converted to medical research and teaching accommodation

1995 UCL Hospitals NHS Trust completed an Outline Business Case to reprovide The Middlesex and UCH hospital services in a new building on Euston Road. The Full Business Case was approved on 12 July 2000

1997 The Bloomsbury School of Nursing and Midwifery was closed

2004 UCLH NHS Trust became UCLH Foundation Trust

2005 The first phase of the new UCH opened to patients and inpatients transferred from The Middlesex to UCH

2006 The Middlesex Hospital island site was sold

References

1 *The Middlesex. Two hundred and fifty years*. A. L. Miller. The Special Trustees. 2005

2 *Our heritage, our future*. UCLH Hospitals NHS Trust. Ronald Mason. 1999

3 *The Middlesex Hospital 1745–1948*. Hilary St George Saunders. Max Parish.1949

4 *A History of Nursing at The Middlesex Hospital 1745–1990*. Monica Baly and Muriel Skeet. The Middlesex Hospital Nurses' Benevolent Fund. 2000

5 *The Middlesex Hospital. The names of the wards and the story they tell*. C. D. Shaw & W.R. Winterton. 1983

The Memories

'The Middlesex had a very tight nursing community. It was a fantastic place to train. Training was very formal – no first names – your hair and uniform had to be just right and no jewellery was allowed. There were no male nurses – it was a bit like a finishing school – many girls came from private schools. There was a tremendous sense of belonging to the hospital. You were very proud of your hospital badge, belt buckle and hat. Life in training was very strict. When you went out you had to roll your sleeves down and put on your cape. When you came back you had to roll back your sleeves and put on your cuffs. Students nowadays are much more diverse and often older and would never have put up with all these rules.'

Sister

'The hospital used to be run by the Superintendent Brigadier Hardy Roberts and Matron Marriot and the two wing sisters. They did a ward round every week and took action on whatever came up!'

Medical student in the 60s and later President of the Royal College of Surgeons

'The commitment of Middlesex nurses to The Middlesex has always been extraordinary.'

Retired Trust Chairman

'The buildings seemed run down and antiquated, which didn't create a very favourable impression – but people's experience of being cared for here were generally so positive that it changed their perception of the building.' ***Voluntary services organiser***

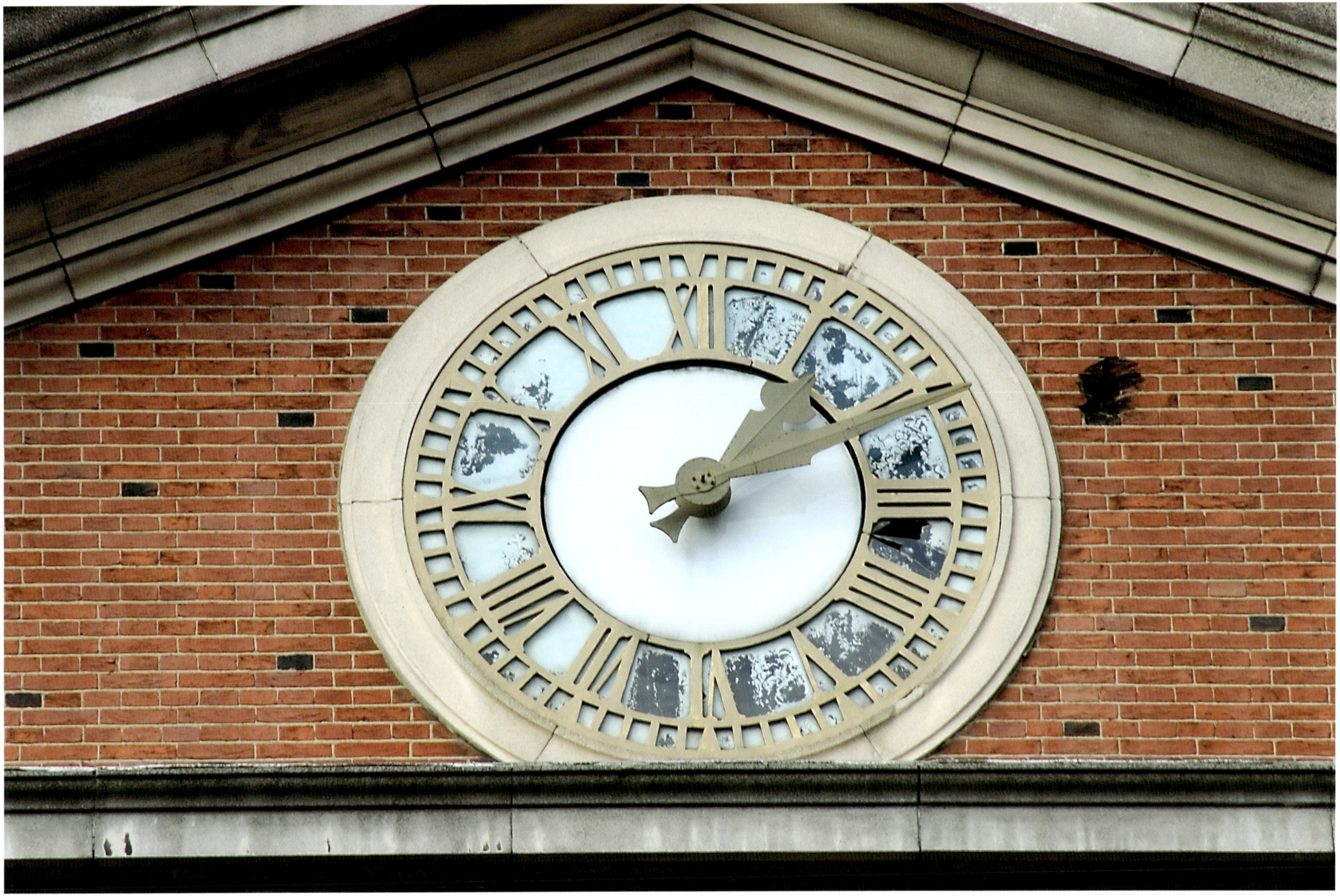

'I was a senior staff nurse in casualty from 1978 to 1980.The casualty department was always busy. It was a beautiful day one Sunday afternoon in 1978, and we were in the nurses home when there was a major incident. Suddenly we were receiving the victims from a grenade and machine gun attack in central London on an El Al bus carrying airline staff. We just dealt with it all and then went home. There was no post traumatic stress counselling in those days. We just did what we'd always rehearsed for. The incident is clear in my mind to this day.'

Sister

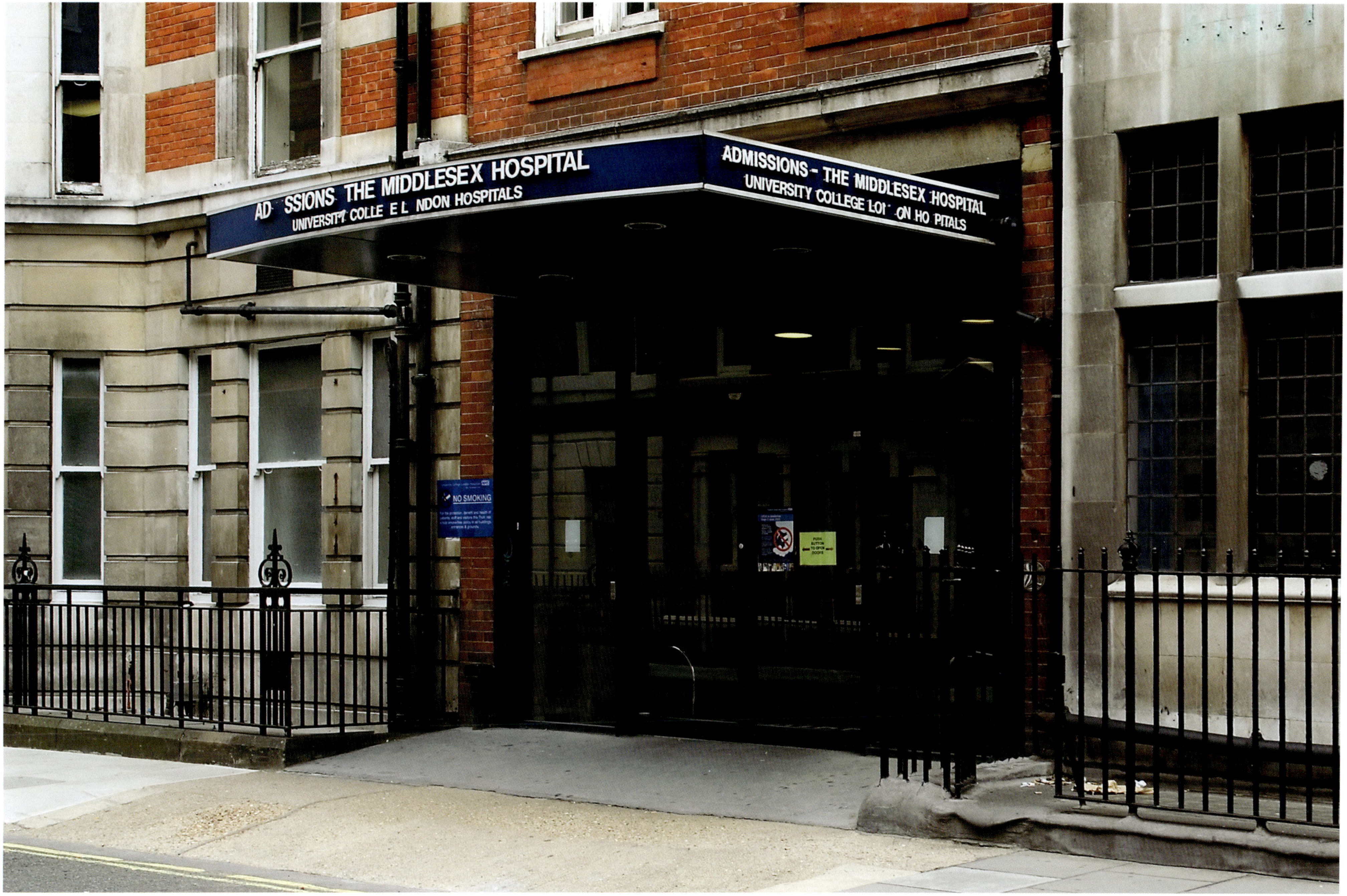
AD SSIONS THE MIDDLESEX HOSPITAL
UNIVERSITY COLLE E L NDON HOSPITALS
ADMISSIONS - THE MIDDLESEX HOSPITAL
UNIVERSITY COLLEGE LO ON HO PITALS
NO SMOKING

'There was an oval polished table in reception which always had flowers on it. In the 80s, it was taken away 'for repairs' by thieves and staff even helped them to unscrew it from the floor!'

Retired orthopaedic surgeon

'There was a real sense of loss following the theft of the oval table in reception – it was somehow a symbol of the quality that The Middlesex provided. There also used to be a name board on the wall so you could see which consultants were in and out.'

Medical student in the 60s and later President of the Royal College of Surgeons

'In the 60s, when the Queen visited the hospital, she was greeted by the head porter wearing a frock coat, tails and a tri cornered hat.' **Nurse who trained in the 50s**

'Sir William Slack, then Dean, once took a group of students through the front reception and asked one of them what the motto meant. He replied 'I learn to make a success out of medicine!'

Retired orthopaedic surgeon

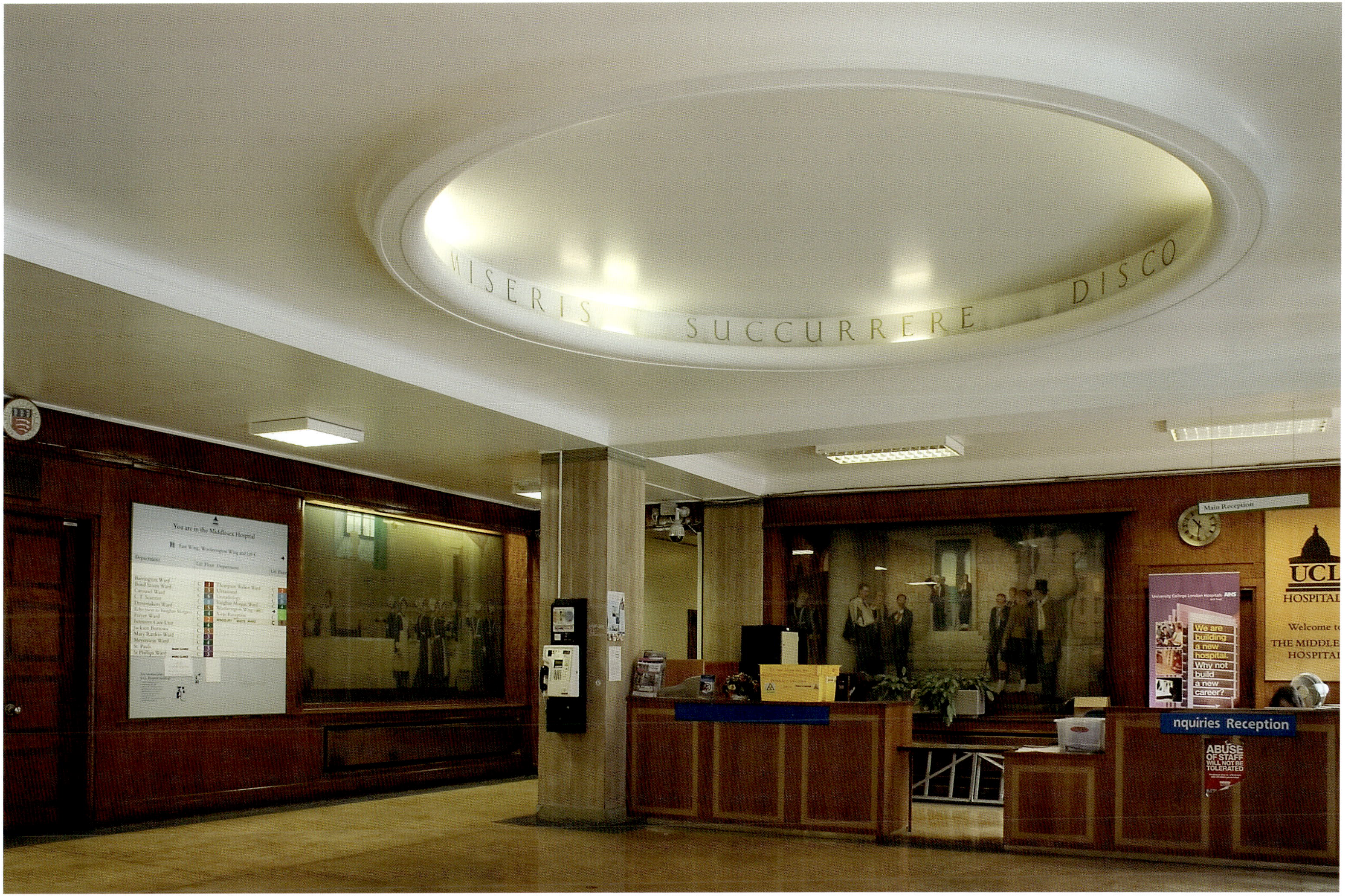
MISERIS SUCCURRERE DISCO
You are in the Middlesex Hospital
Main Reception
We are building a new hospital. Why not build a new career?
nquiries Reception
ABUSE OF STAFF WILL NOT BE TOLERATED

'The Middlesex was a very warm, friendly and tight knit community. The reception area and long central corridor were important meeting places and helped people to communicate.' **Nurse consultant ICU**

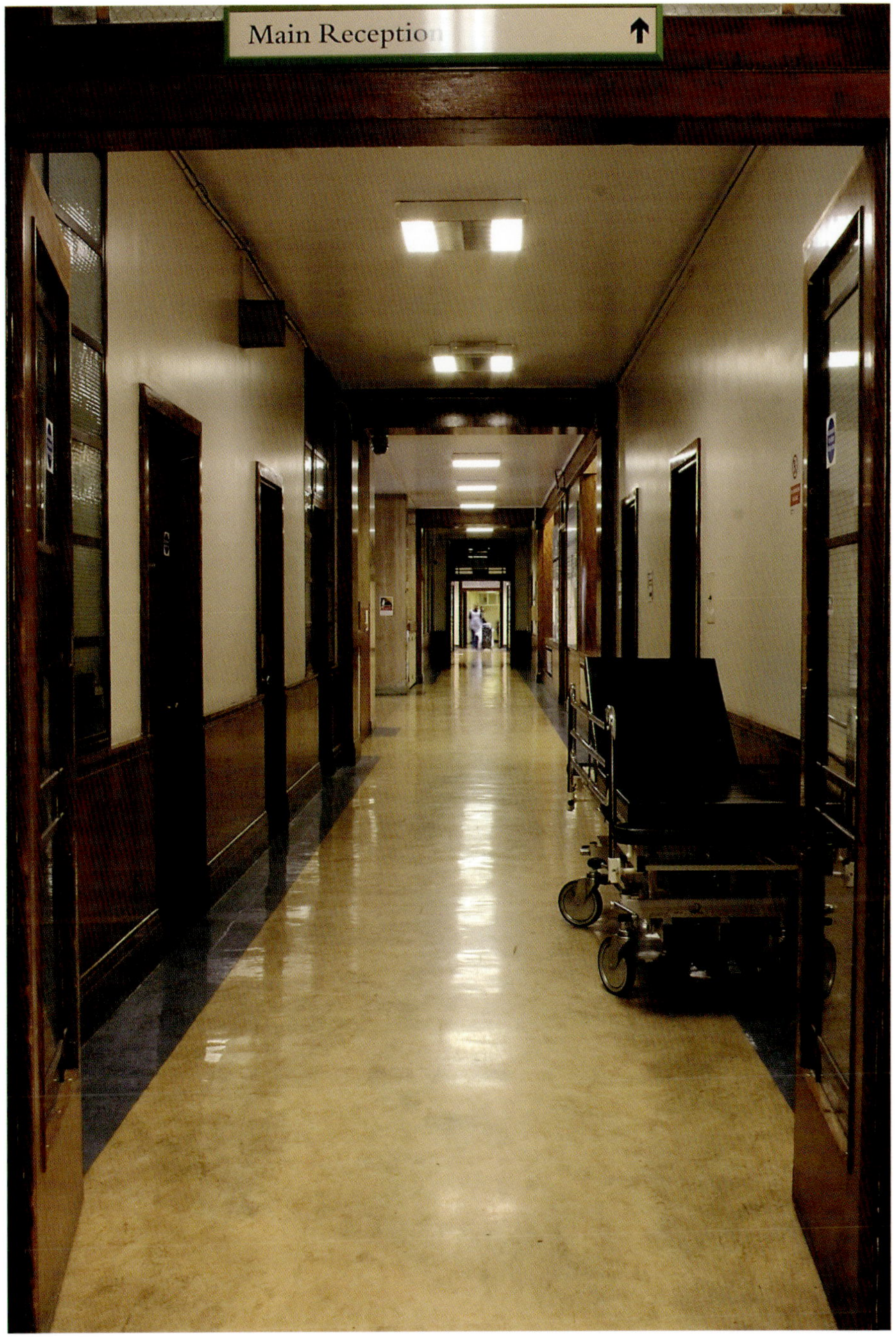
Main Receptio

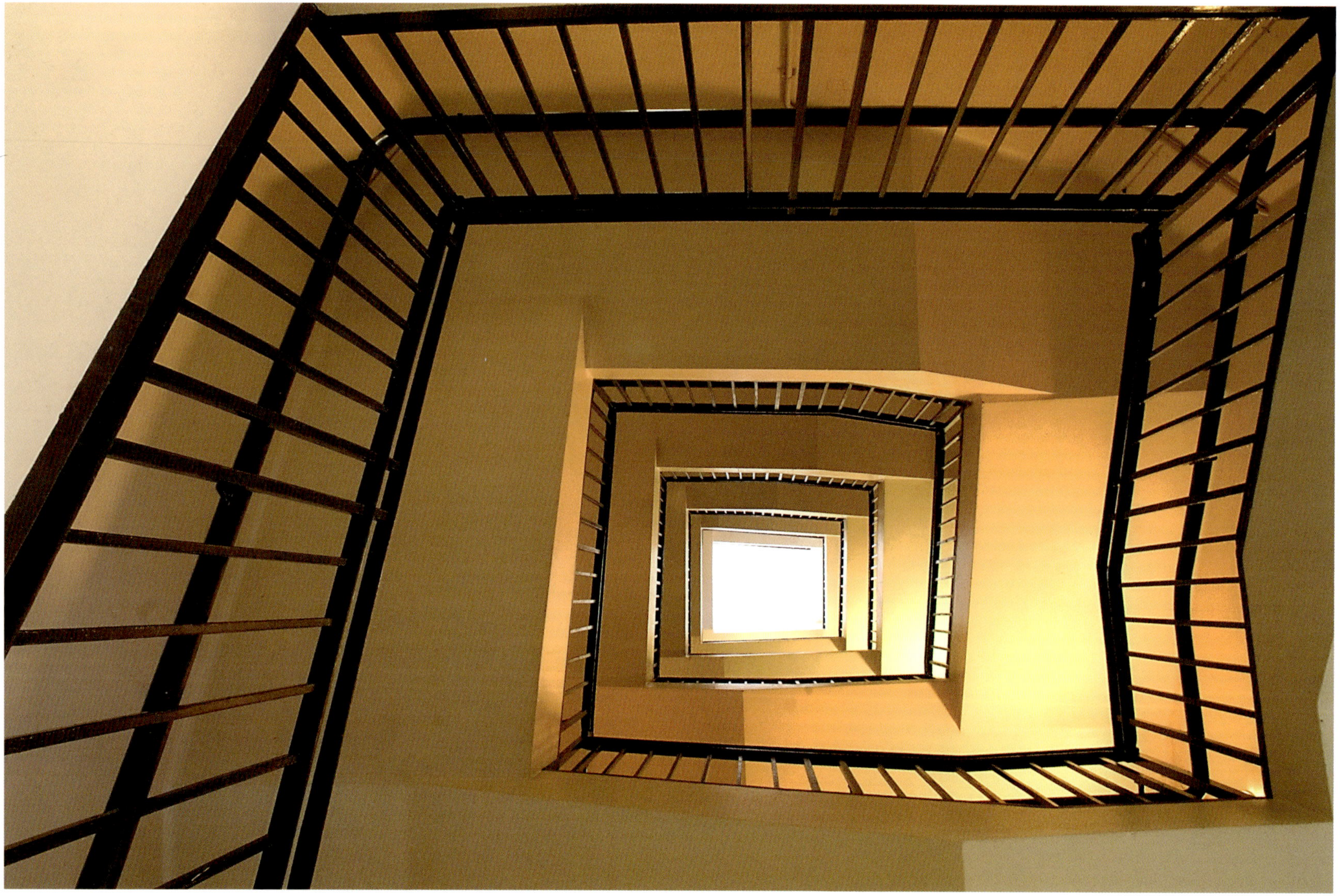

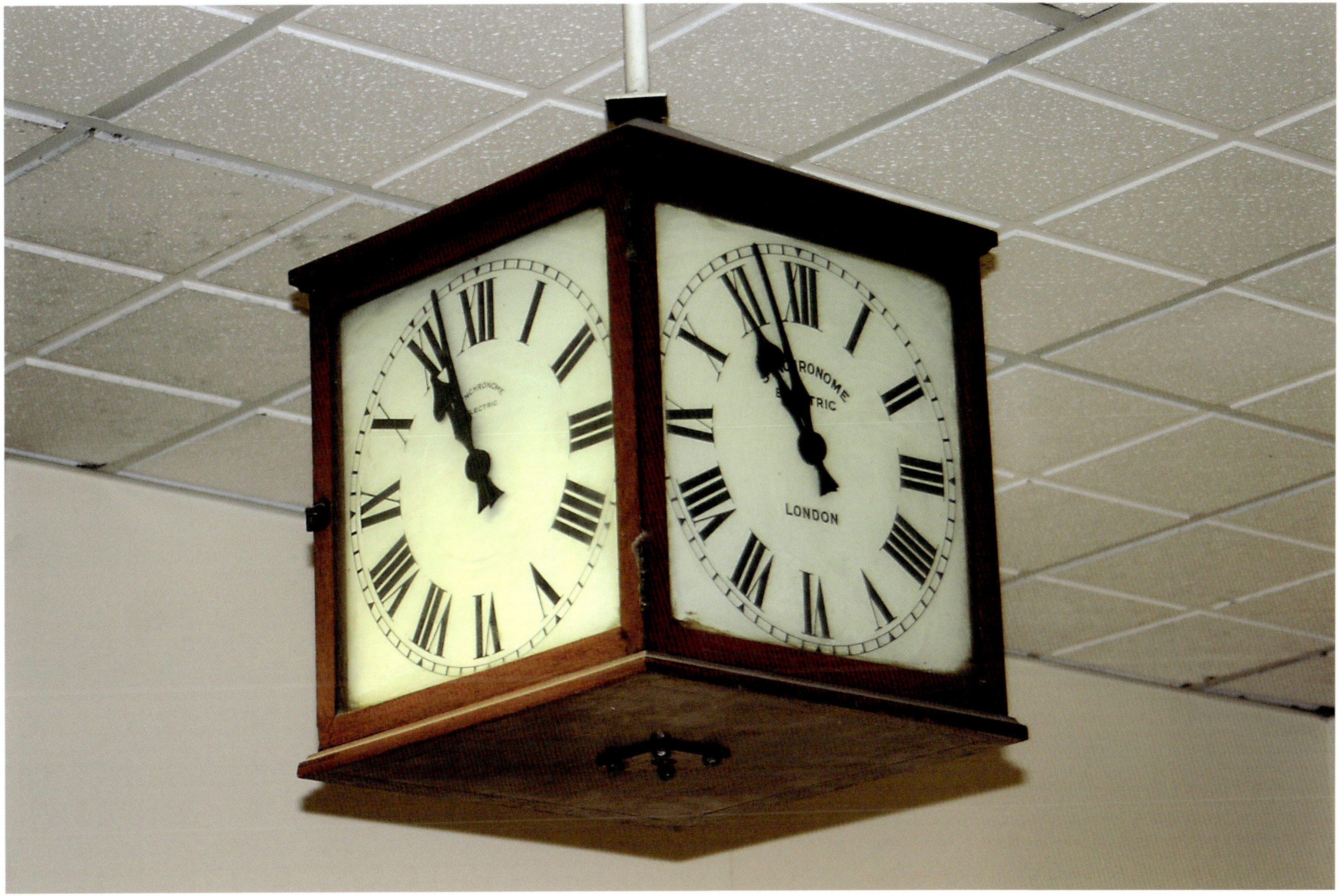
LONDON

'Lord Astor sat in the Chairman's high chair at Board meetings. There used to be a large oval polished table in the boardroom which was also used as the consultants' lunch room, where they were waited on for a three course silver service lunch and got a bill once a month.' **Past member of the Board**

'Interviews with the Medical Committee were held in the Boardroom and could be very intimidating. The Chairman sat in the Chairman's chair – any consultant could attend and ask you about anything.'
Retired surgeon

'The Boardroom was a regular meeting place for consultants at lunchtimes – they were a tight knit community and many clinical problems were discussed and resolved over lunch.' **Retired surgeon**

'Night sisters and staff nurses used to sit in state in the Boardroom at night. We thought this was an amazing experience. People using it nowadays don't realise how special it felt for nurses to be there in those days.' **Sister**

'I certainly remember the Boardroom clock – Health Authority meetings started at 5 o'clock and we were often still here at 10 o'clock still struggling to take difficult decisions on budgets and cuts.'
Member of Bloomsbury Health Authority in late 80s

'Lots of open meetings to discuss the new hospital PFI project were held in the Boardroom – protestors came by the busload and created absolute chaos – meetings had to be closed.' **Retired Trust Chairman**

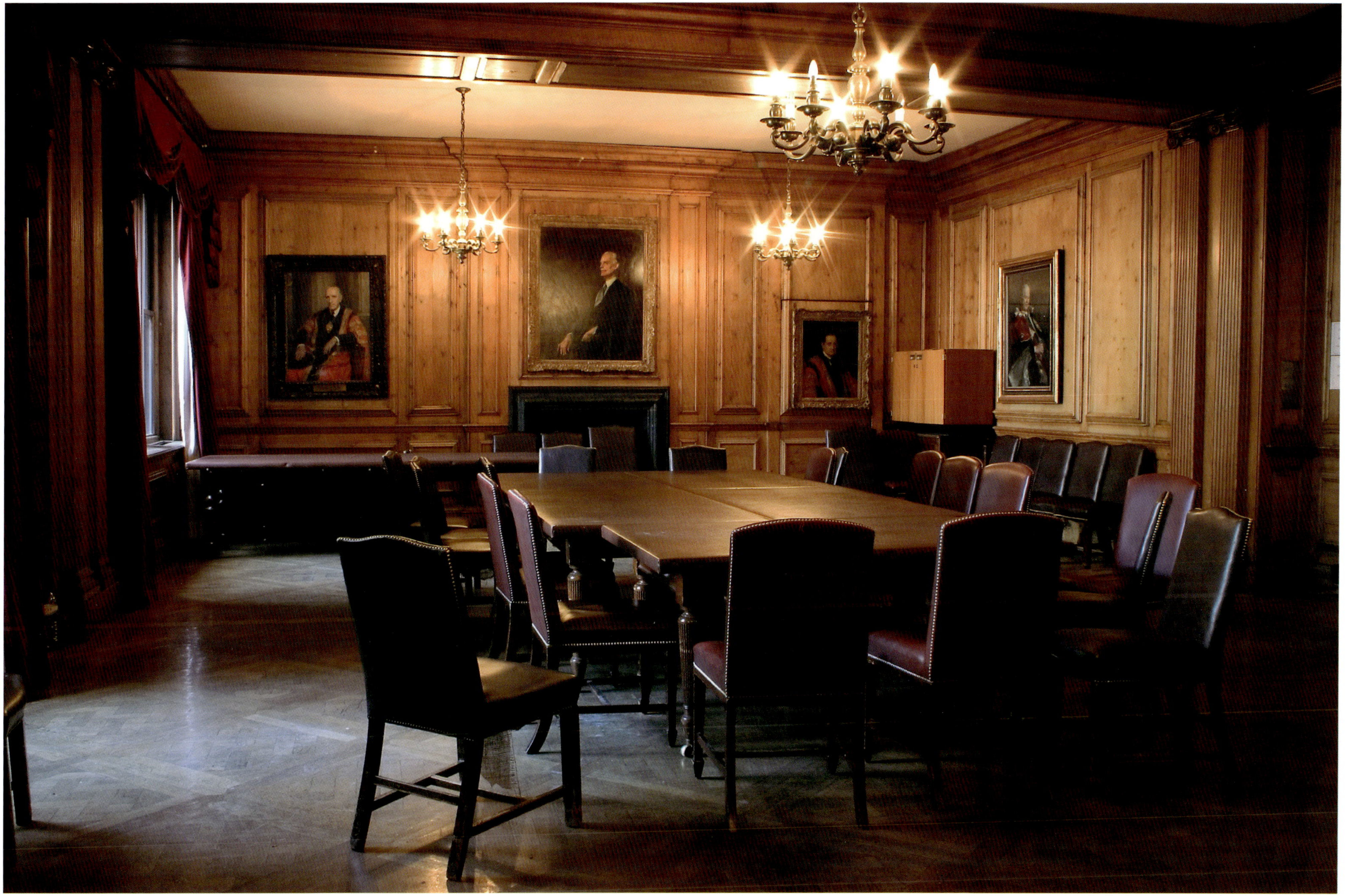

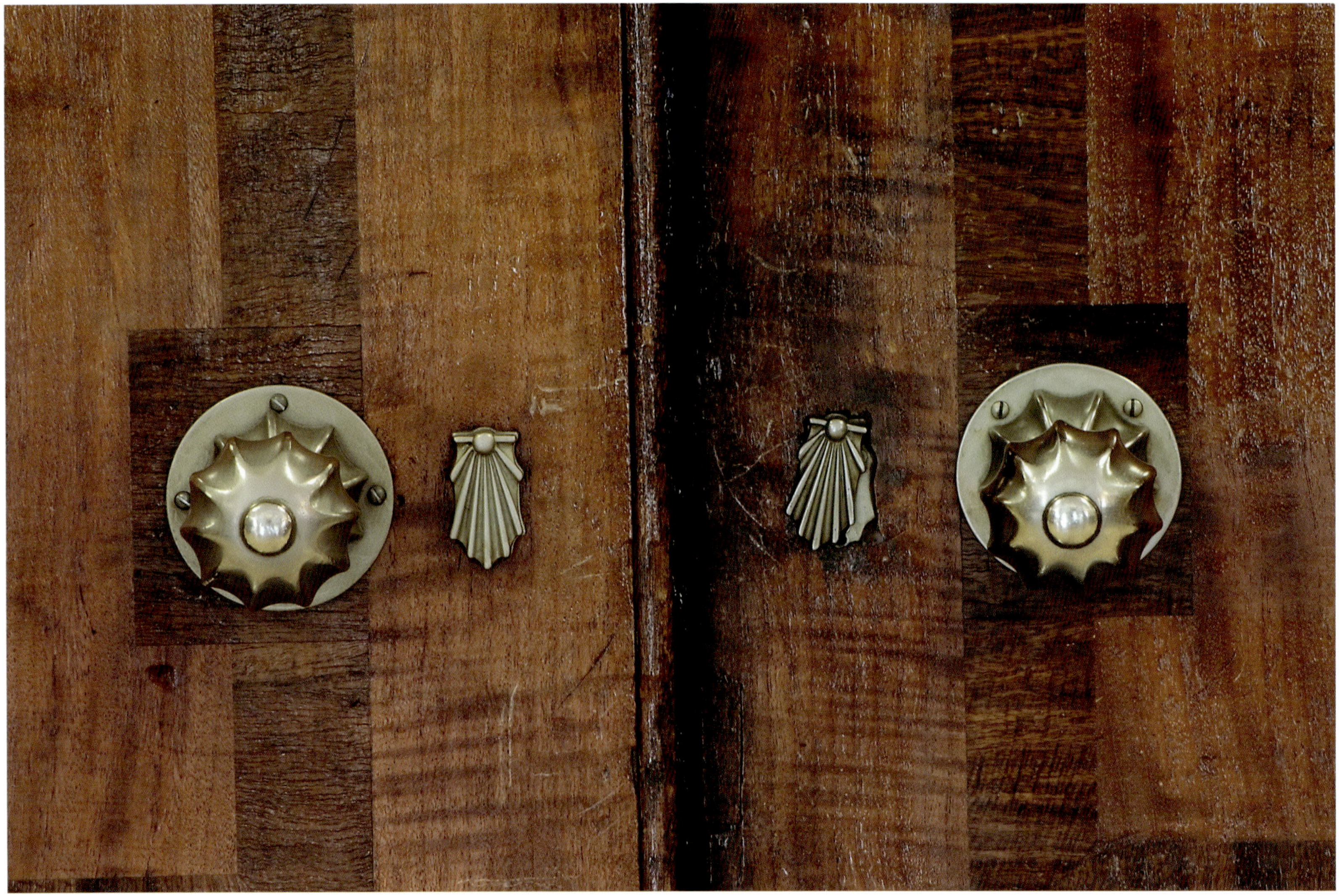

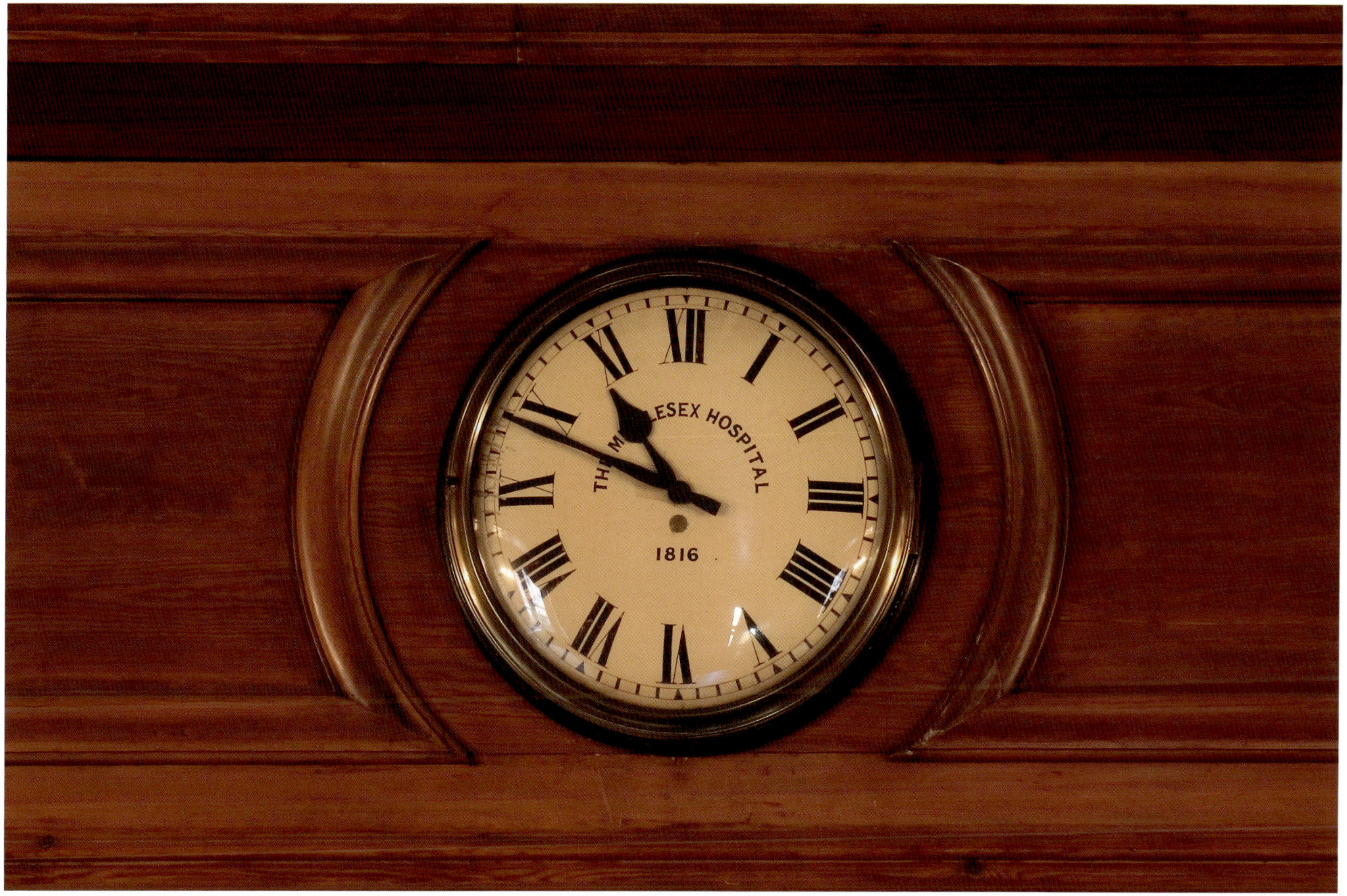
THE M LESEX HOSPITAL
1816

'The Chapel has been used for memorial services for staff – some of the memorial plaques go back a long time and are part of the Chapel's history. Because the Chapel is a separate building from the hospital, it is possible for people to light candles here – something that is often important to many people. The blue mosaic work in the baptistery is very special and has been offset to create the ripple effect of water.'

Chaplain

'The Chapel's central position in the hospital has been very important – people could just drop in when they had bad news to cope with or difficult decisions to make.' ***Retired surgeon***

'I remember the Chapel at Christmas, it would be all lit up, with night lights around the top and the font – it looked wonderful.' ***Senior nursing officer who trained in the late 40s***

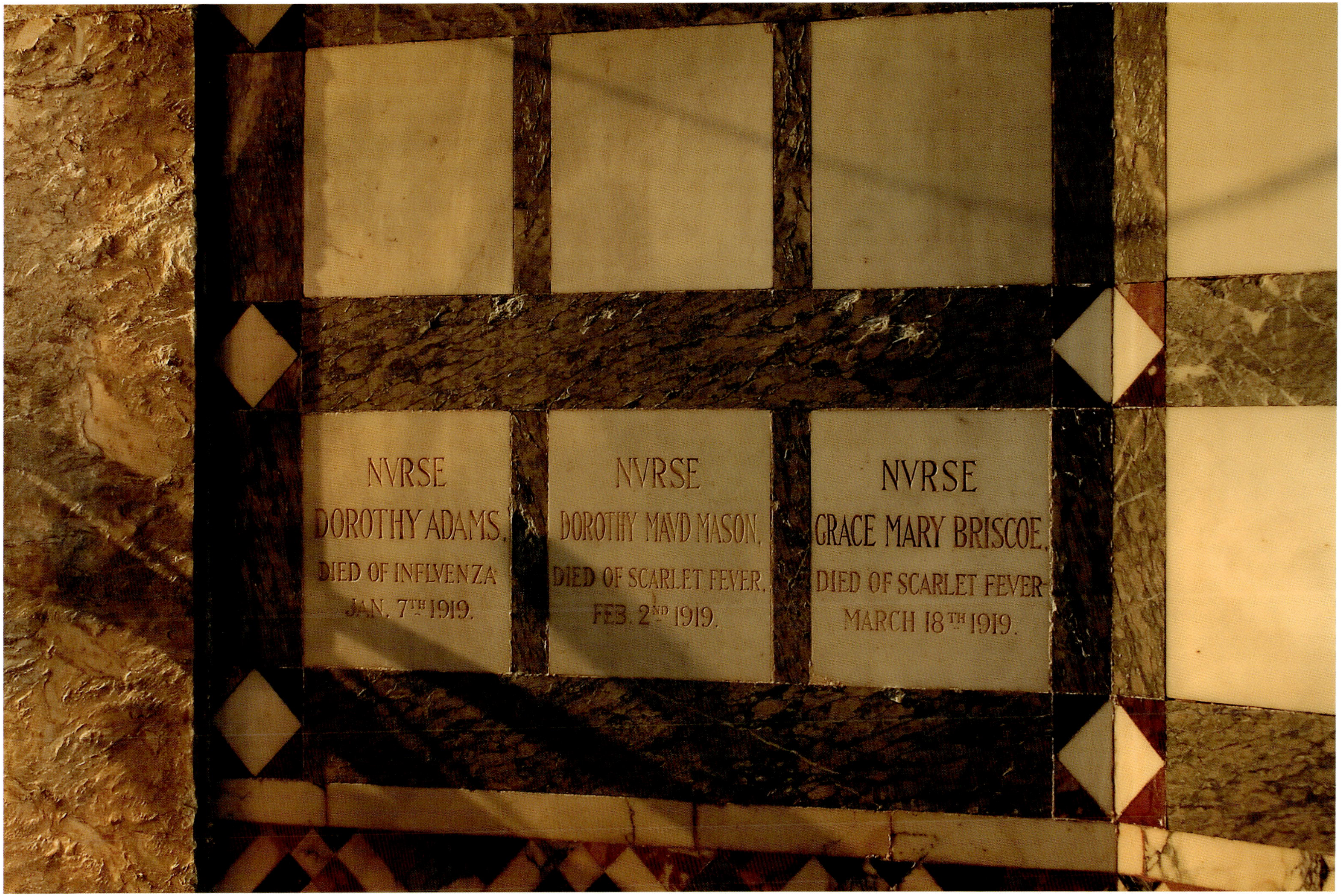
NVRSE
DOROTHY ADAMS.
DIED OF INFLVENZA
JAN. 7TH 1919.
NVRSE
DOROTHY MAVD MASON.
DIED OF SCARLET FEVER.
FEB. 2ND 1919.
NVRSE
GRACE MARY BRISCOE.
DIED OF SCARLET FEVER
MARCH 18TH 1919.

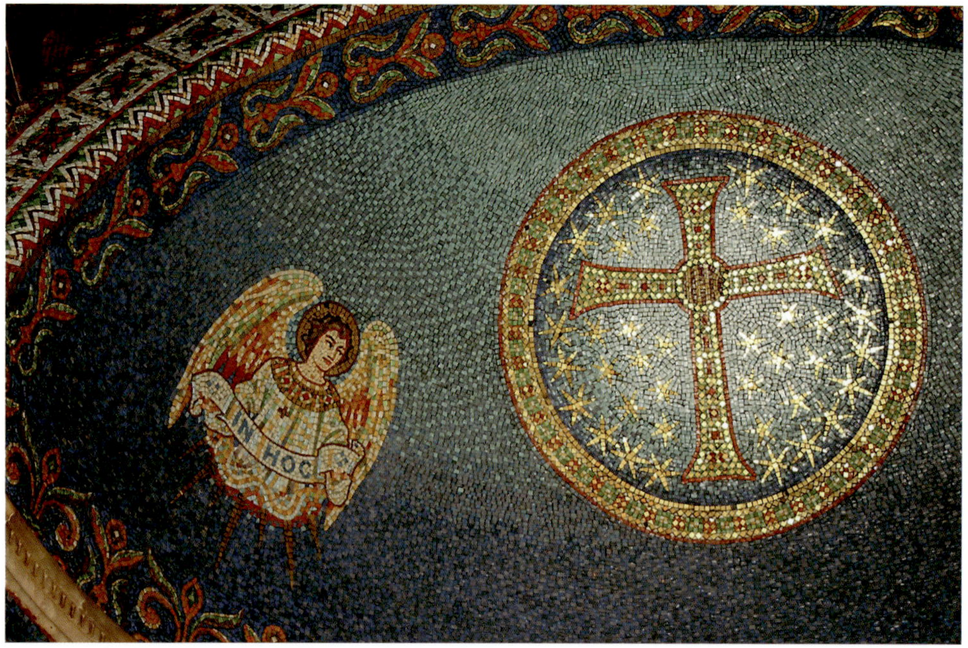
IN HOC

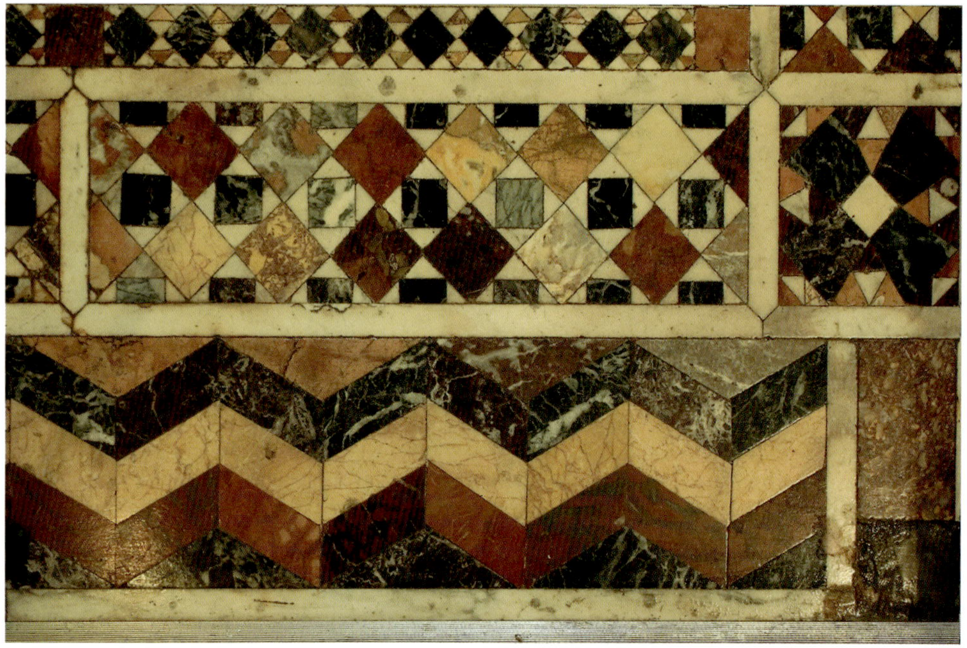

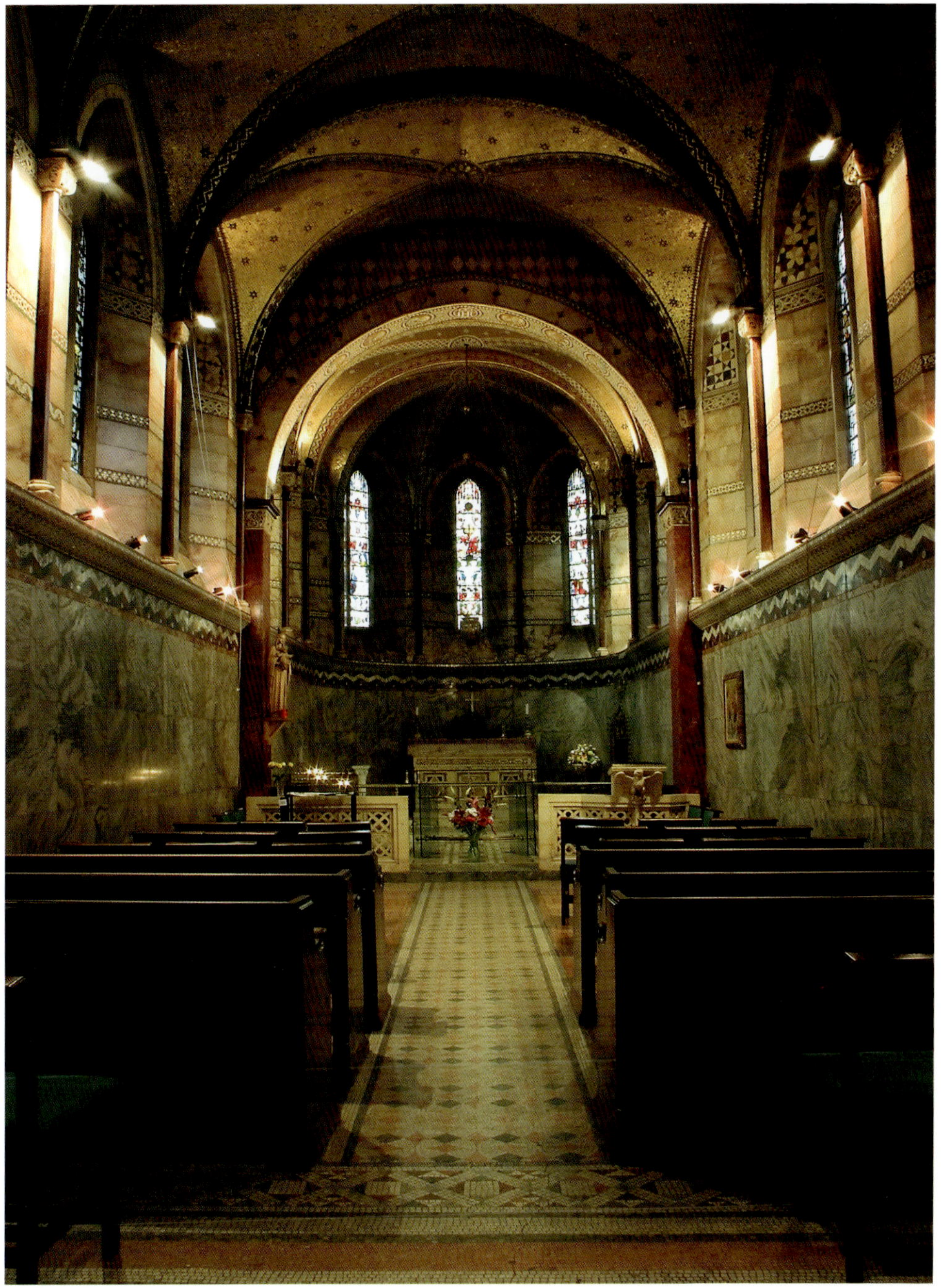

*'The sub basement was used to store all kinds of equipment –
it was a very creepy area.'* **Nurse consultant ICU**

'The sub basement used to be the operating theatres in World War II.' **Head porter**

'This was a ghostly eerie place' **Retired clinical service manager**

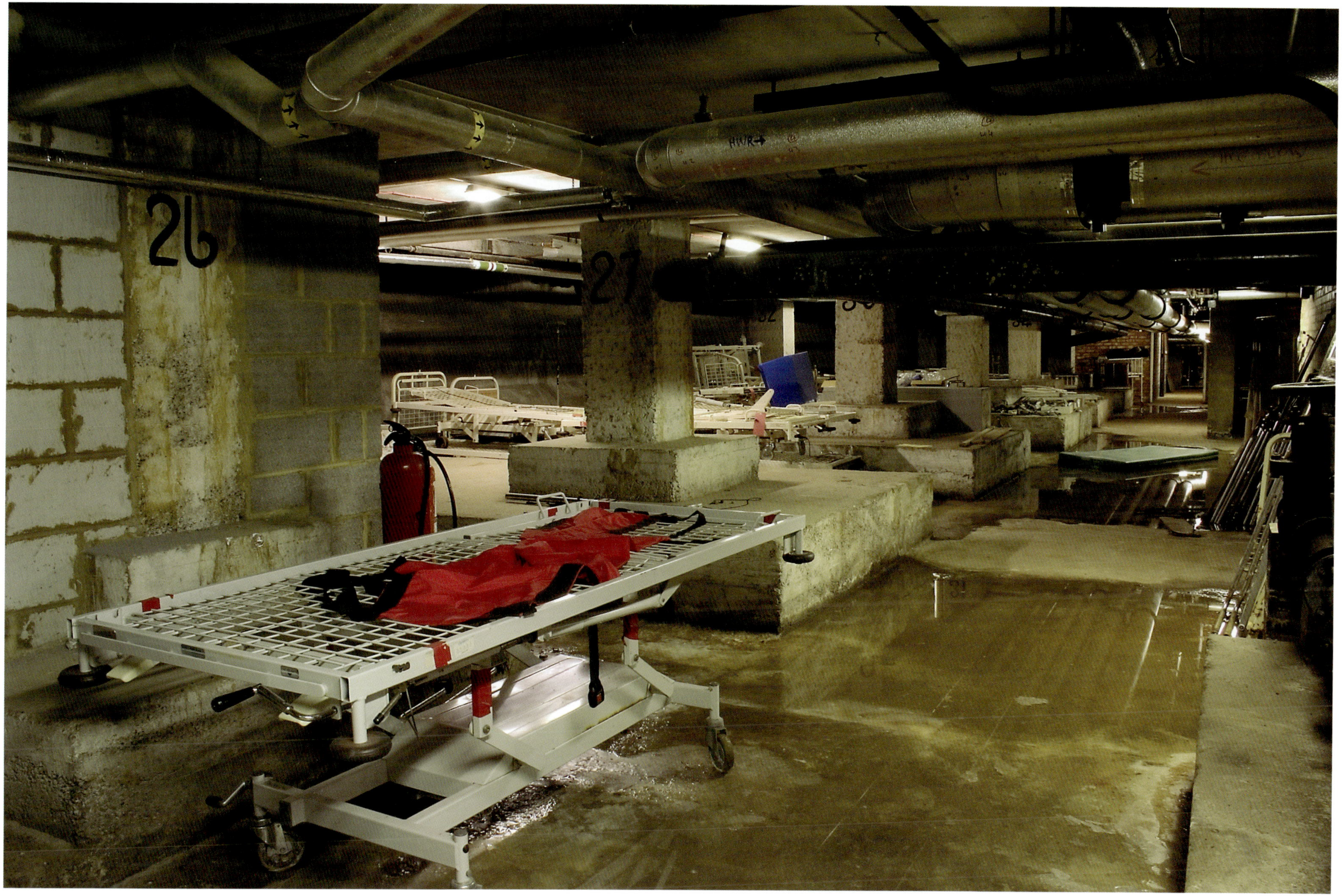
26
27

'This used to be the dining room for a small residency for medical students who lived in for one week in four and for doctors in residency. The latter didn't earn much but were well looked after. A maid cleaned your room upstairs, a man on the door cleaned your shoes and three meals a day – all paid for – were served in the dining room. Matron looked after the residency.'

Retired surgeon

'Above what is now the SNAX bar, medical students and doctors used to live in – celibacy for students and doctors was strictly enforced by matron who sat in the room below.'

Medical student in the 60s and later President of the Royal College of Surgeons

'What's now the SNAX area used to be out of bounds to nurses. After an arsonist attack on the hospital, security wouldn't supply staff at night without hot food being available – so it was provided for nurses and doctors on duty as well. It was such a luxury to have hot evening meals instead of cold vending machine food.'

Sister

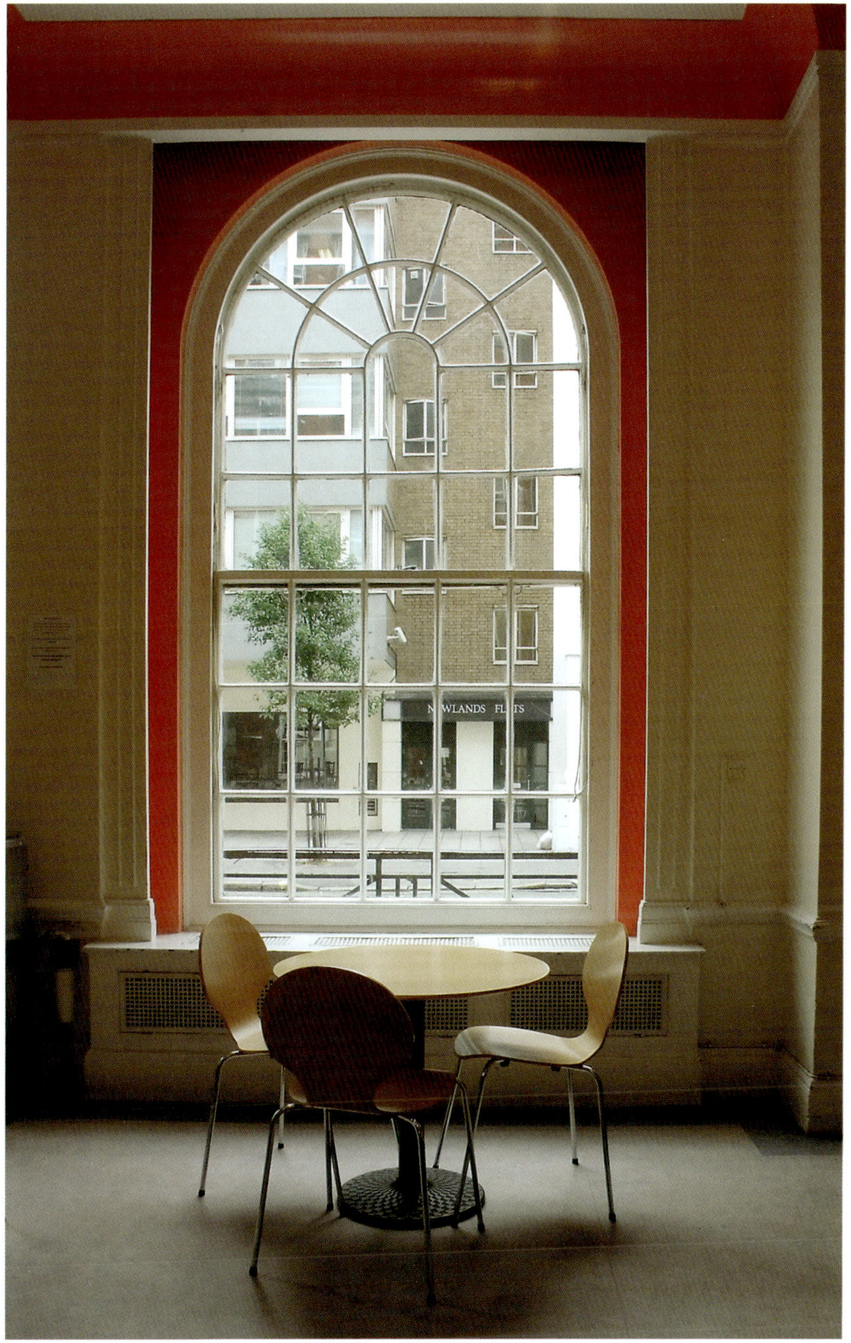

'Specimens for biopsy from sixth floor theatres used to travel through the air from the sixth floor across the courtyard garden to the pathology institute on a little rail system like a mini cable car – results were then telephoned back to the theatres.'
Retired orthopaedic surgeon

'After the Christmas parties for staff children organised by 'Mrs Mouse', the children would go on tours around the hospital. The group that went to theatres, all equipped with hats, masks and overshoes were very impressed by what went on in there.'
Radiotherapy consultant

'The Woolavington theatre had natural light and daylight – very important to surgeons – this is where Churchill had his hip done.'
Medical student in the 60s and later President of the Royal College of Surgeons

'The Day Surgery Unit used to be the orthopaedic department and before that housed the main operating theatres for the hospital. There is a plaque commemorating Sister Thomas who, in 1934, was awarded the George Cross for her bravery in extinguishing a burning oxygen cylinder in an anaesthetic room. Philip Whiles, a senior orthopaedic surgeon devised and carried out the first hip replacement in this department.'
Past President of the Royal College of Surgeons

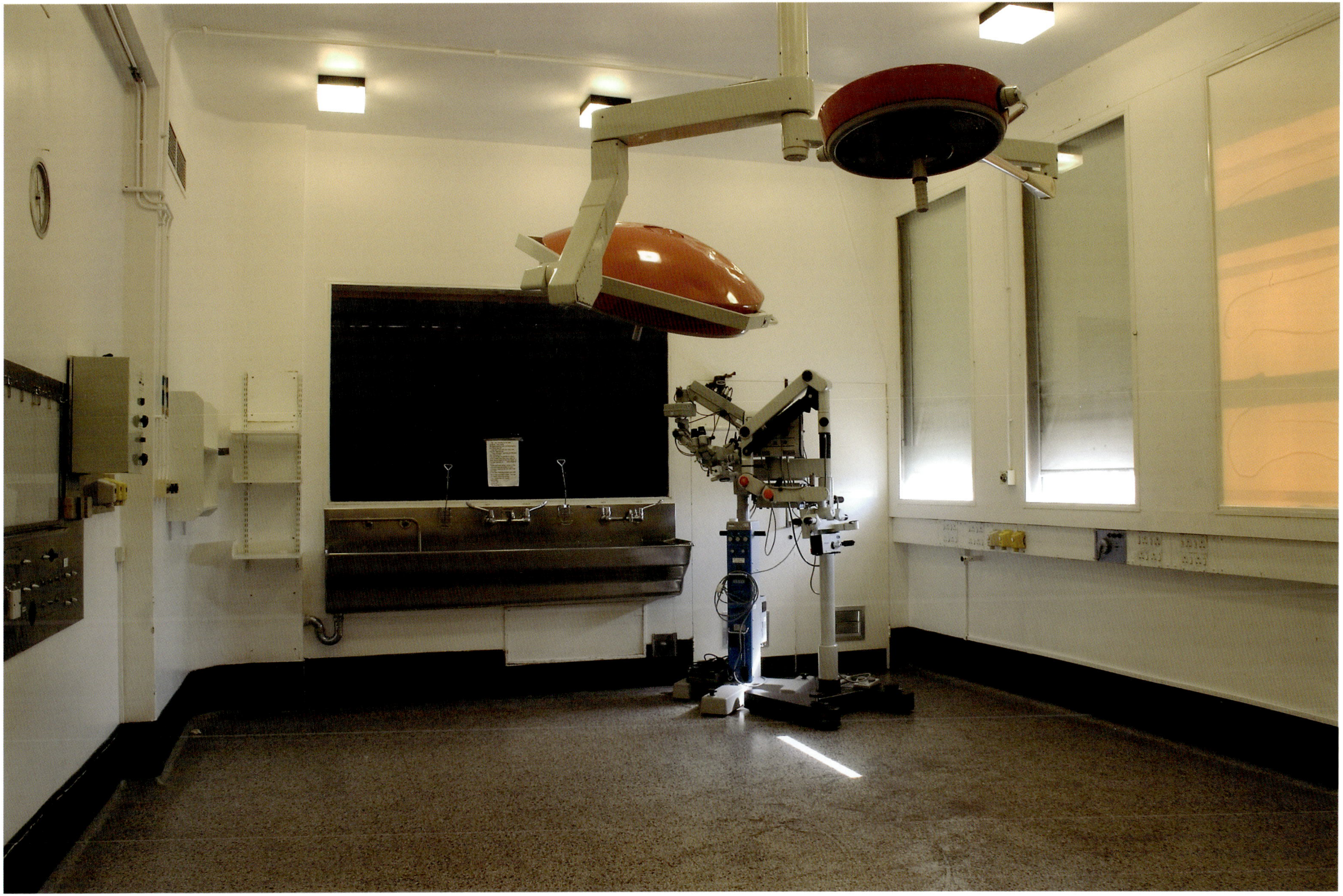

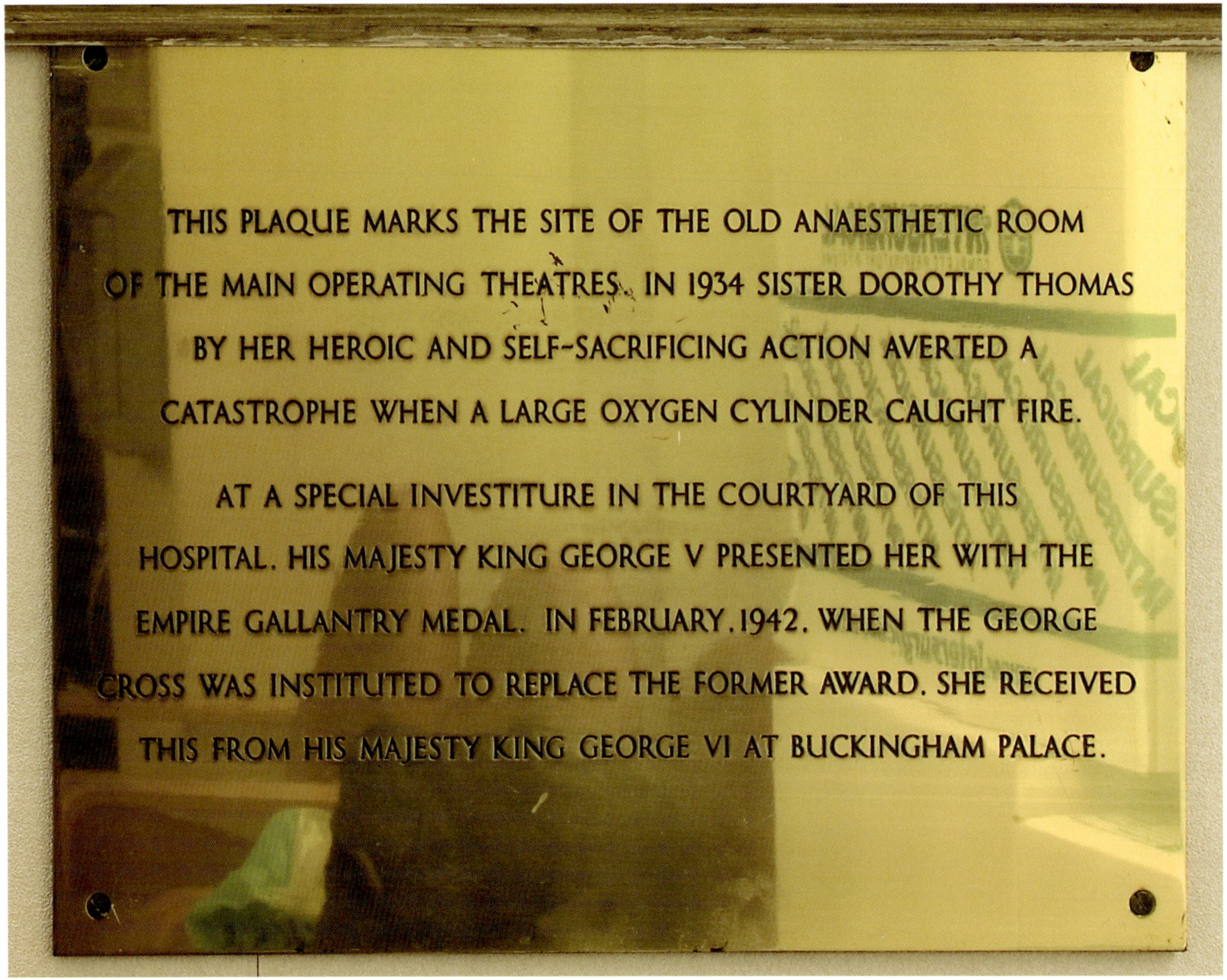
THIS PLAQUE MARKS THE SITE OF THE OLD ANAESTHETIC ROOM
OF THE MAIN OPERATING THEATRES. IN 1934 SISTER DOROTHY THOMAS
BY HER HEROIC AND SELF-SACRIFICING ACTION AVERTED A
CATASTROPHE WHEN A LARGE OXYGEN CYLINDER CAUGHT FIRE.
AT A SPECIAL INVESTITURE IN THE COURTYARD OF THIS
HOSPITAL. HIS MAJESTY KING GEORGE V PRESENTED HER WITH THE
EMPIRE GALLANTRY MEDAL. IN FEBRUARY. 1942. WHEN THE GEORGE
CROSS WAS INSTITUTED TO REPLACE THE FORMER AWARD. SHE RECEIVED
THIS FROM HIS MAJESTY KING GEORGE VI AT BUCKINGHAM PALACE.

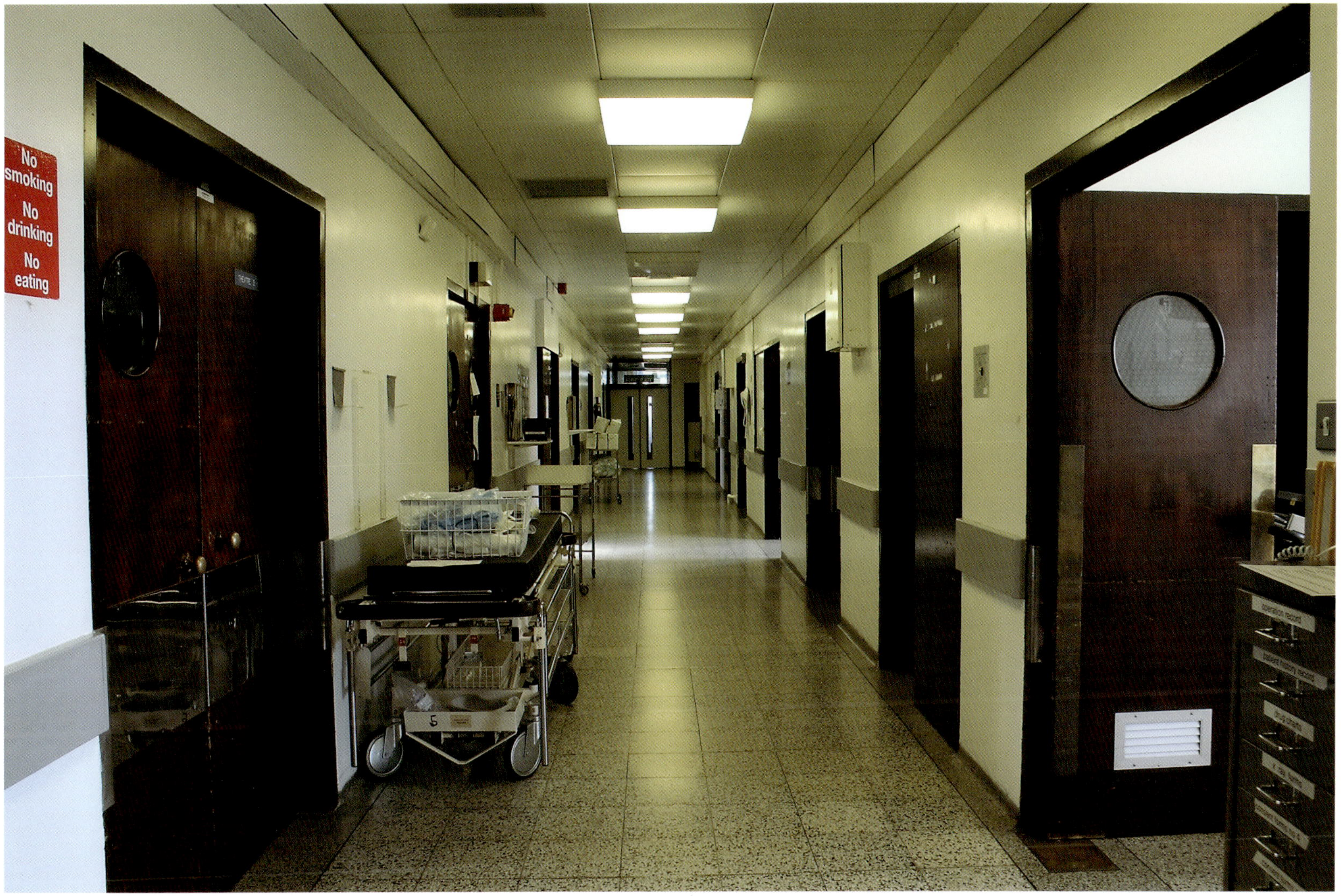
No
smoking
No
drinking
No
eating
operation record
patient history record
drug charts

'What was unusual about The Middlesex was the close integration of teaching, research and the hospital – all on one site.' **Retired surgeon**

'The Courtauld lecture theatre was the hub of teaching in the hospital – David Patey gave a demonstration of cases at 4pm every Friday. Situated in the centre of the hospital, it had medical and surgical wards on either side.' **Retired surgeon**

'A great thing about The Middlesex was the cross fertilisation of ideas between physicians and surgeons. This was helped by the central location in the hospital of the Courtauld lecture theatre where grand rounds were held involving different specialties. The consultant lunches in the Boardroom were also good for cross fertilisation of ideas.' **Retired orthopaedic surgeon**

'I appeared in front of a conference of doctors in this big lecture room. The senior doctors talked about my shoulder to the younger doctors and discussed among themselves what should be done. It was quite an experience. Afterwards they said it was best to leave it alone.' **Patient**

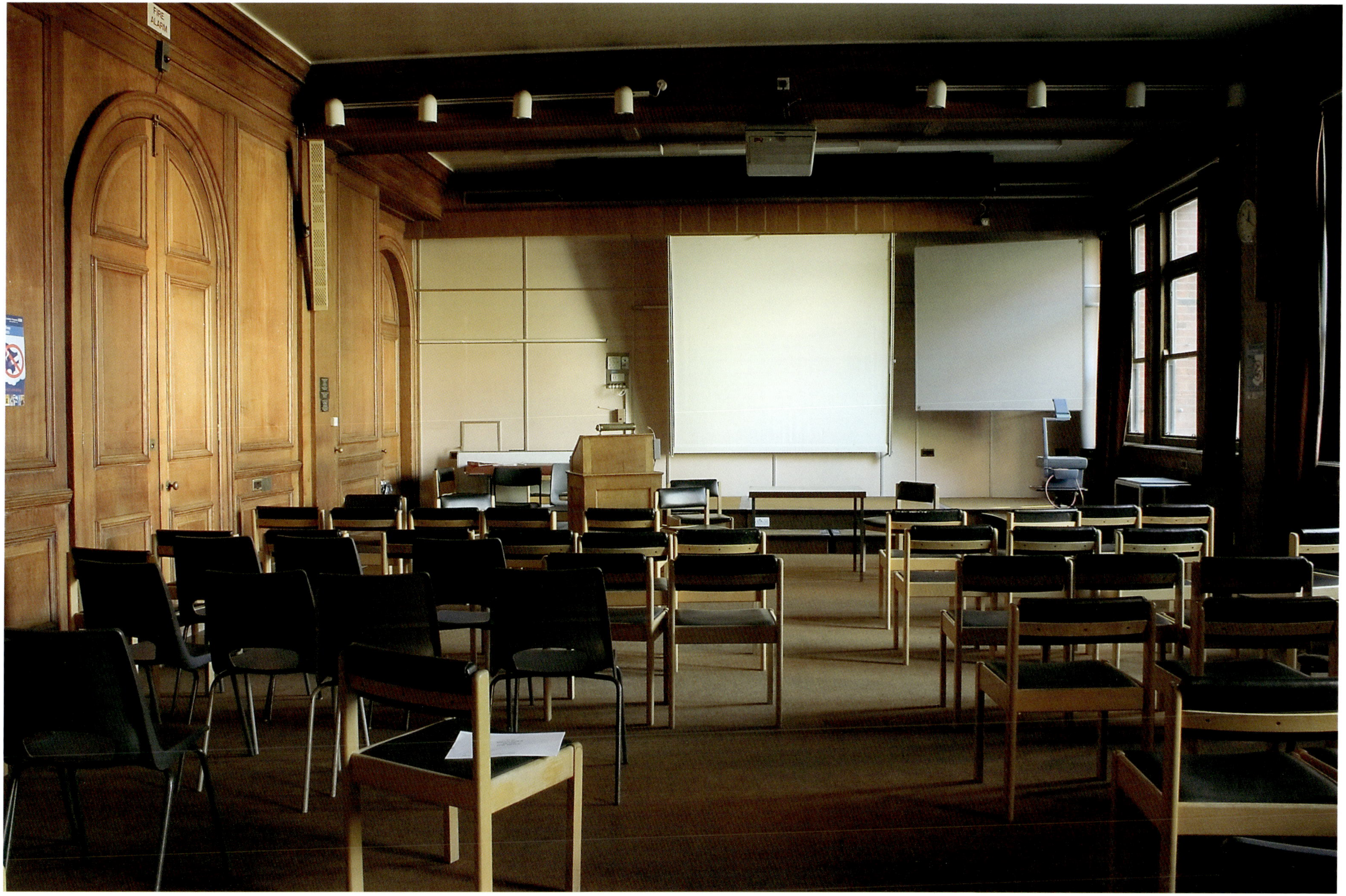
FIRE
ALARM

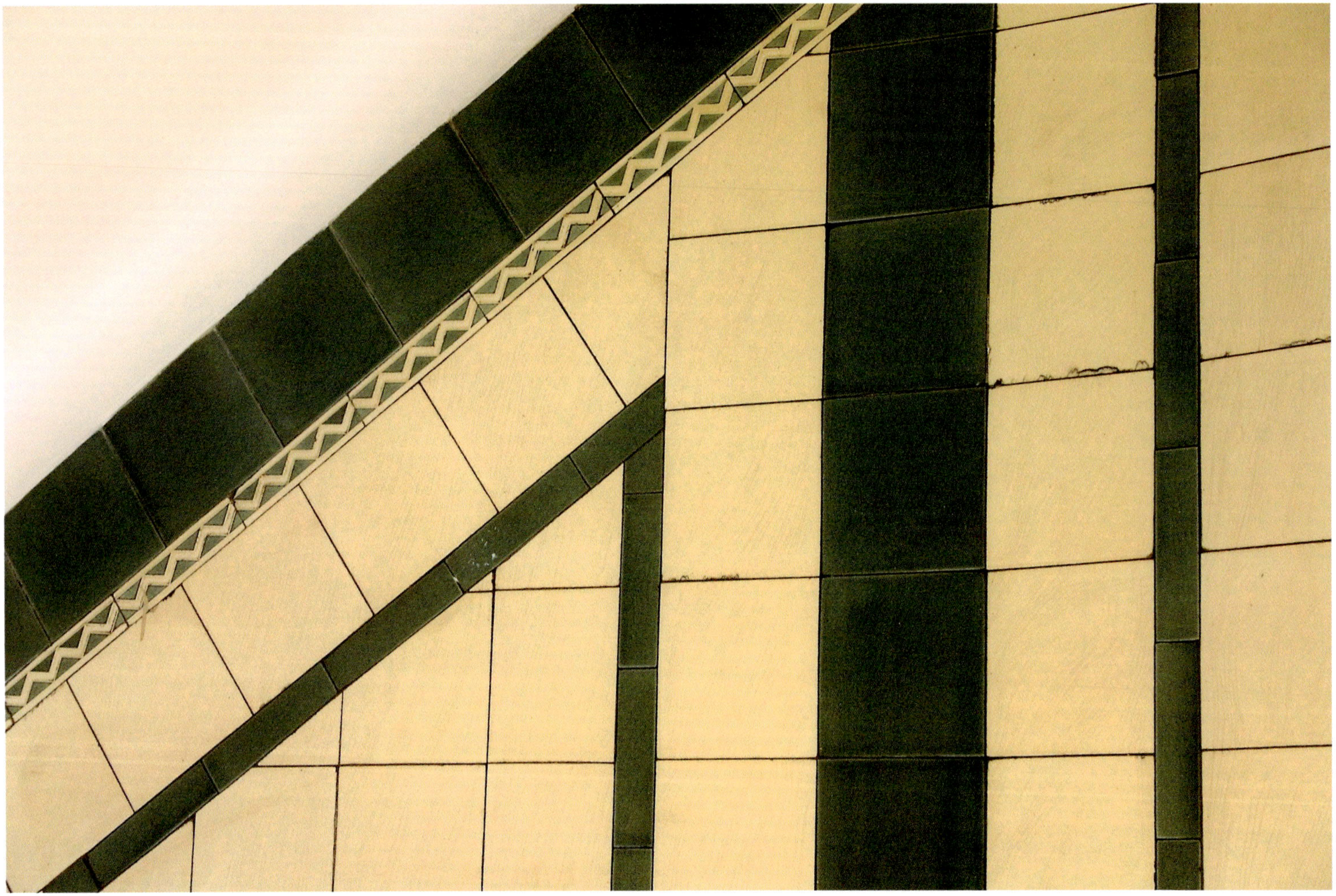

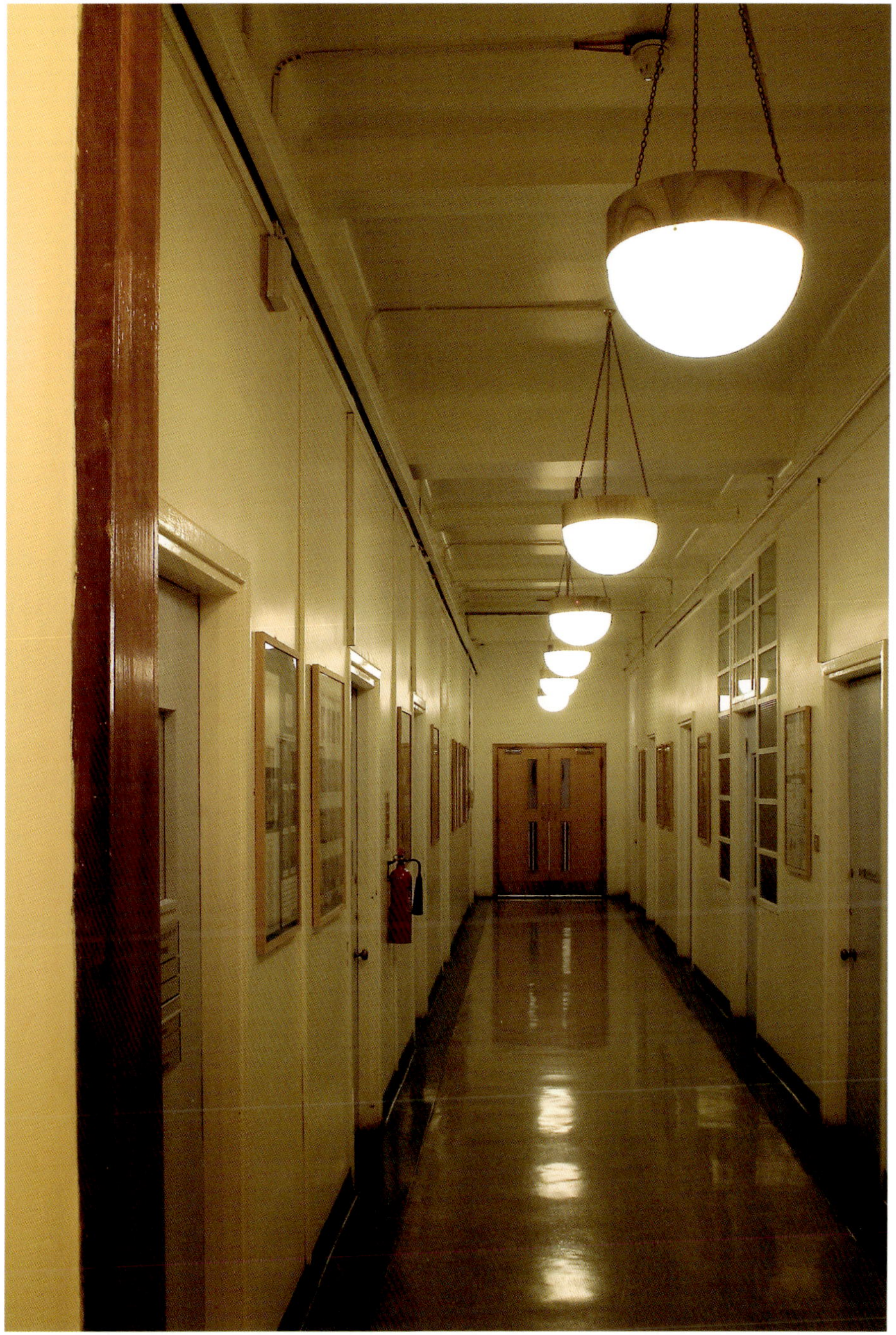

'Drew Thompson, a Senior Lecturer in the 50s and 60s had a huge skill for teaching pathology. He held people totally spellbound.'

Retired surgeon

'The Bland Sutton Theatre was a super room where wonderful pathology lectures were held – it was hard to remain unnoticed there – particularly if you were late.'

Medical student in the 60s and later President of the Royal College of Surgeons

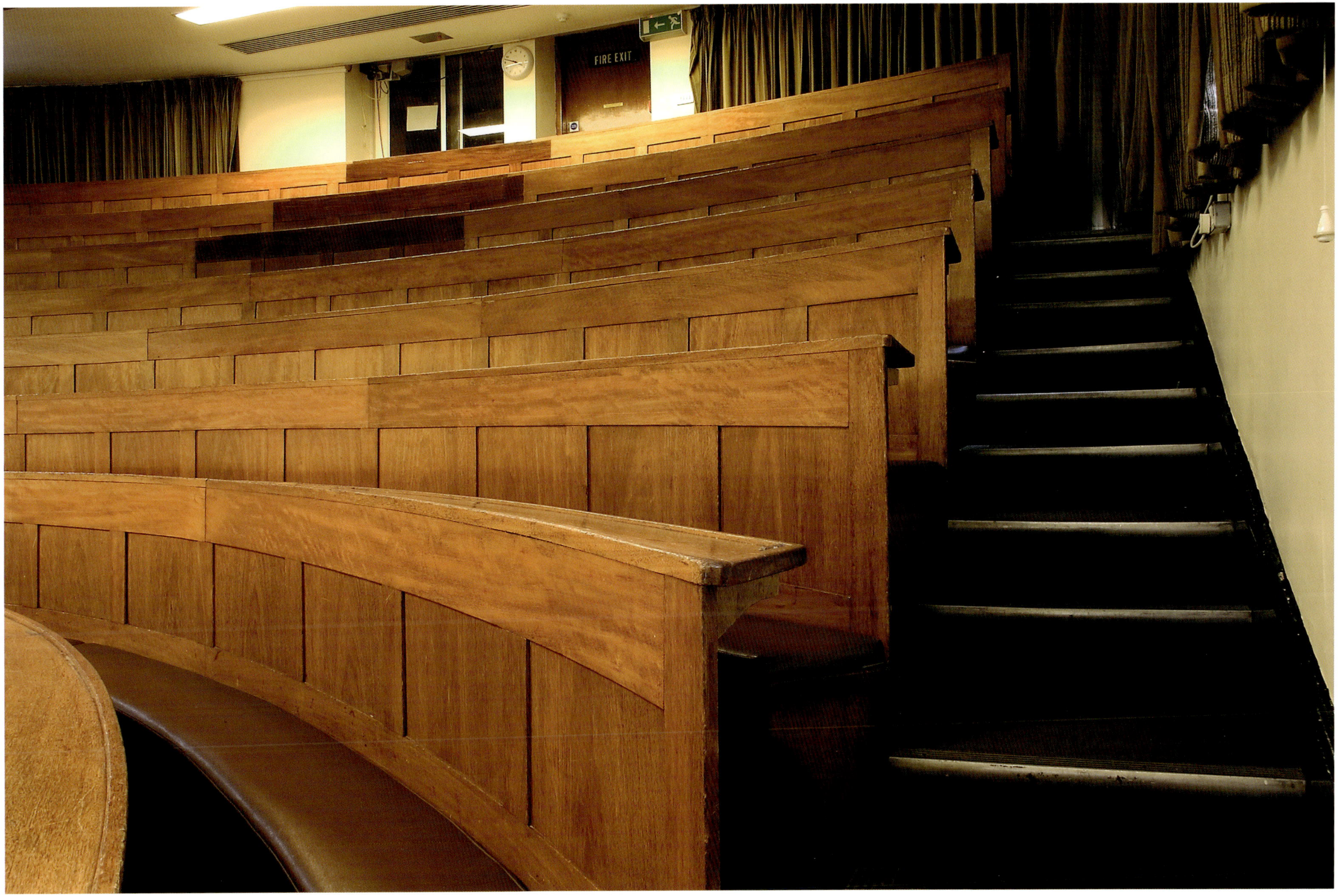
FIRE EXIT

'I also loved the underground corridors where you could pop out in another part of London altogether.'

Nursing student on placement in 1982

'There used to be rumours of a ghost in the basement – underneath the BJ wing. One night a charge nurse came to see the night sisters in the Boardroom looking as white as a sheet saying that someone dressed in white had tried to strangle him.'

Retired clinical service manager

'You could hear trolleys in the basement that you never met'

Past Chair of the League of Friends

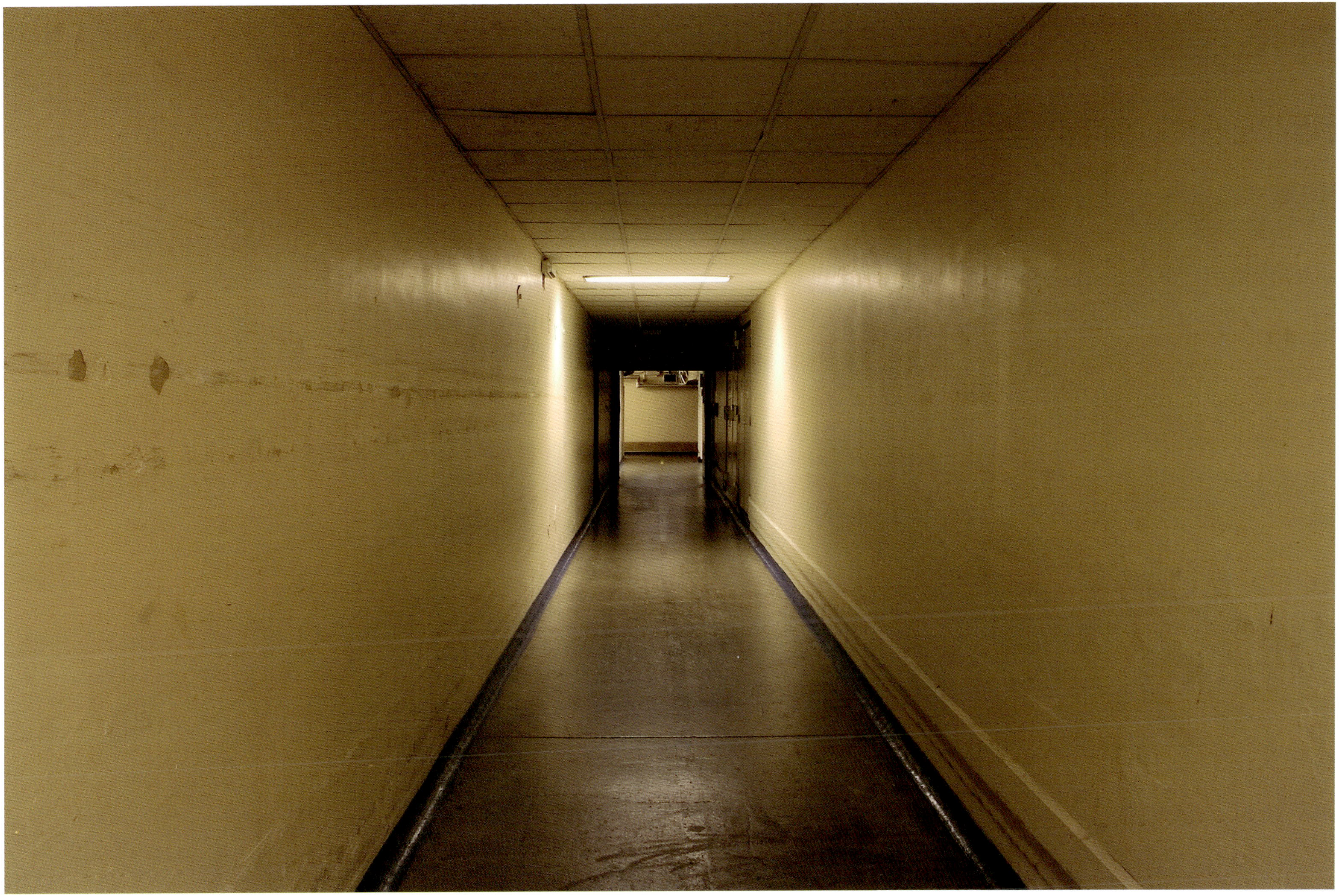

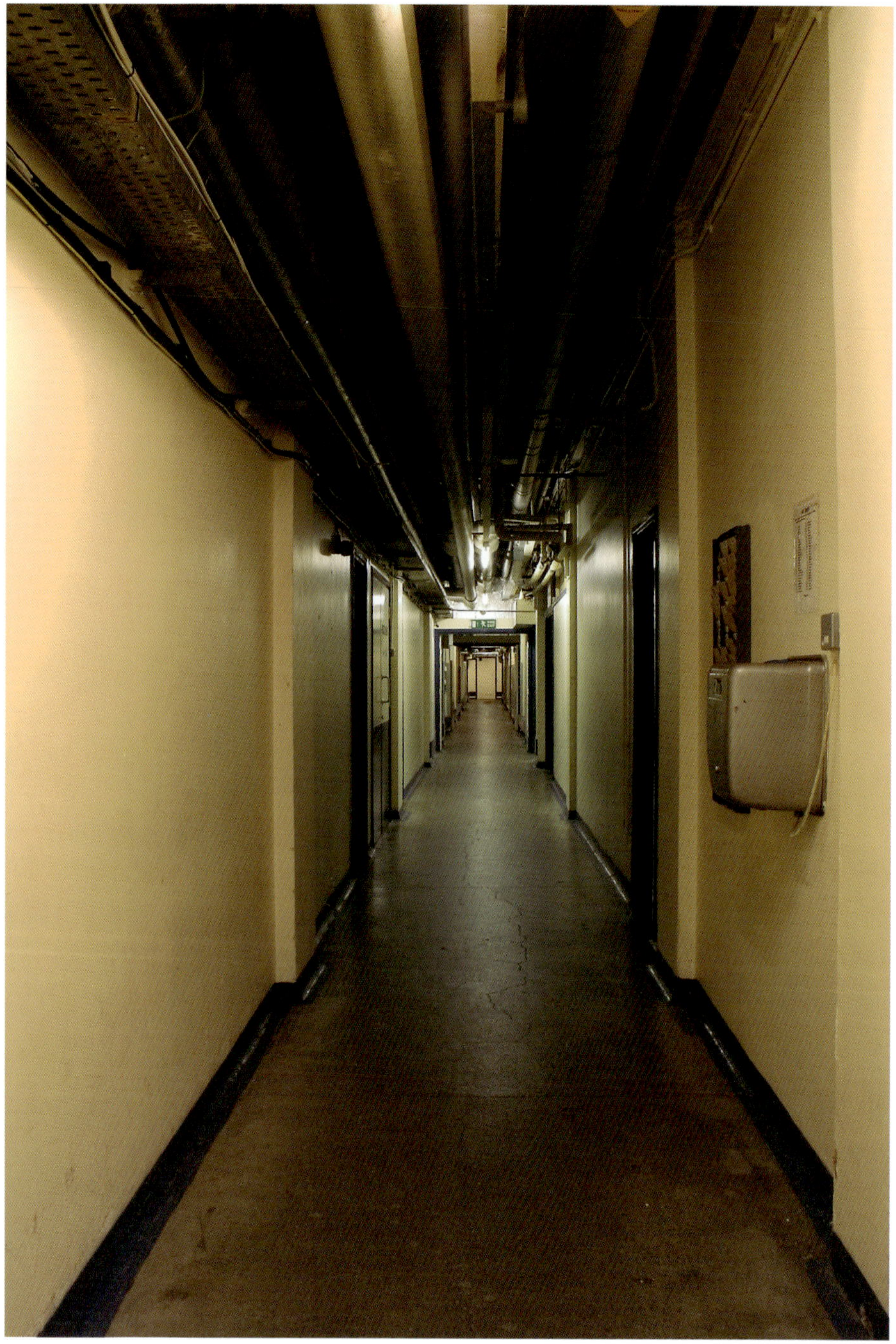

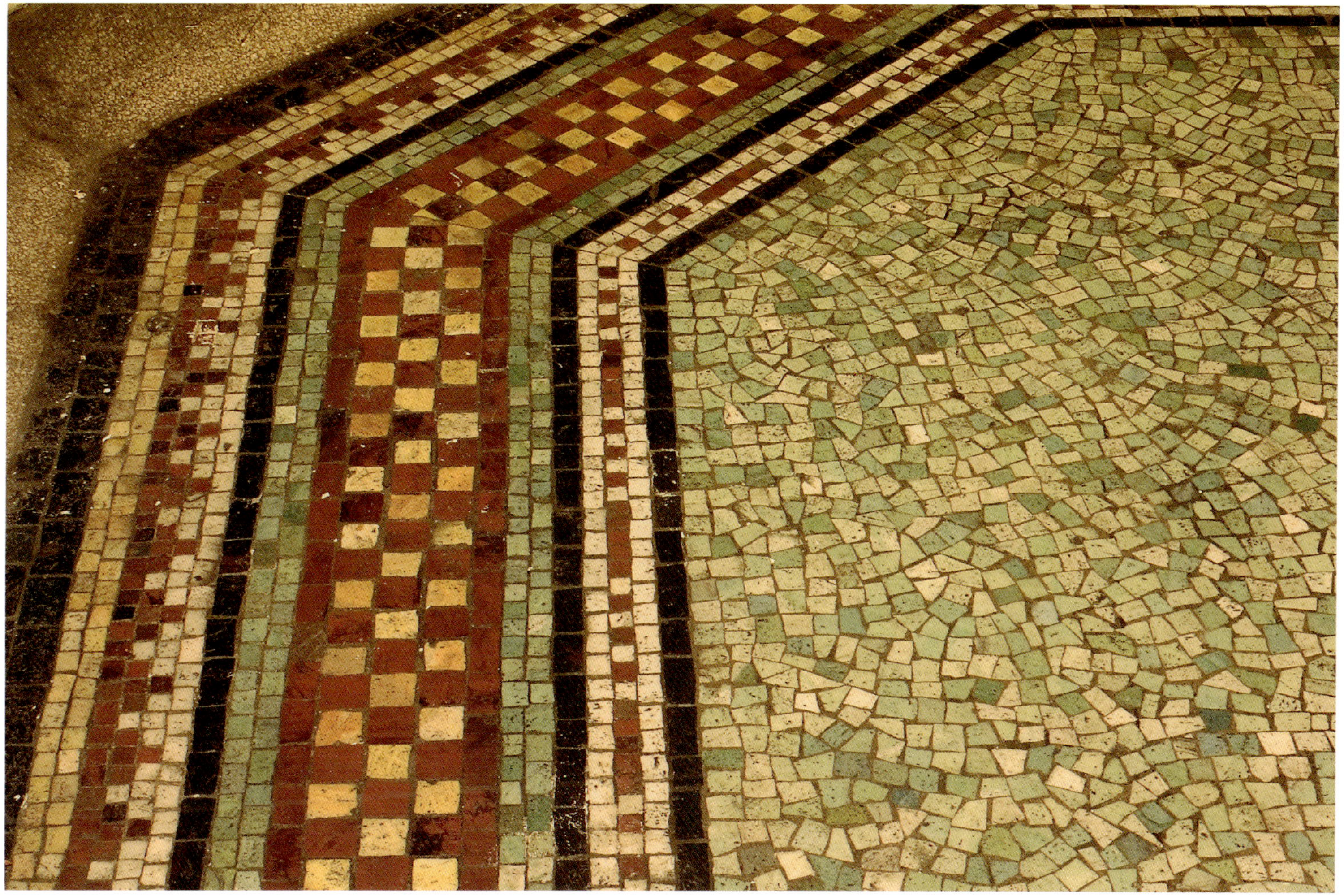

'Breakfasts for patients used to be prepared on the wards by the night staff. The first year day staff would squeeze out the tea leaves till dry and then sprinkle them under the patients' beds – the tea leaves picked up the fluff and dust from the blankets and were then swept up so that the domestics could mop the floors. second year nurses dusted lights and bed tables.

On night duty we also used to sew surgical swabs – called dabs – for use in the operating theatres. We would pick up a list of what sizes were required when we went to the dining room for our meal break.

Brigadier Hardy Roberts, the superintendent, and Matron Marriot did weekly ward rounds and took instant action on any issues that came up.

On Christmas Eve after all the raucous parties outside, the hospital withdrew into itself. Nurses sang carols on the wards and turned the lights down to give atmosphere. Brigadier Hardy Roberts who lived in a house on Cleveland Street, next to outpatients, used to invite sisters to his house on Christmas Eve for champagne and smoked salmon sandwiches.' **Sister who trained in the 50s**

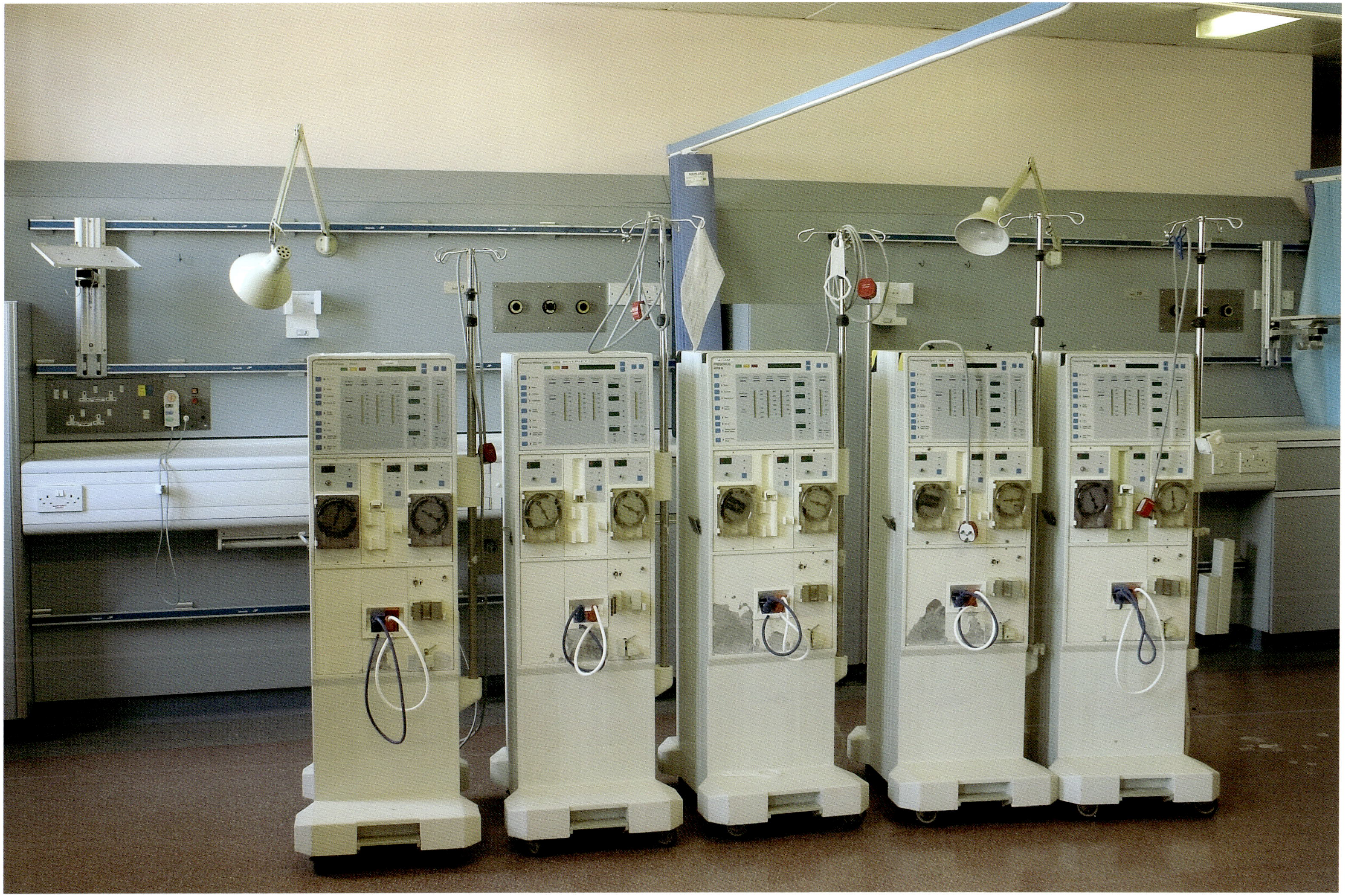

'I was a patient on this open ward in the late 60s. Other patients said that once your bed started being moved towards the door, you were really on your way out. This was partly true as sicker patients were kept by the nurses' station which was at that end.' **Patient**

'The open wards like Bland Sutton all used to have large heaters in the middle to keep the ward warm.'
Medical student in the 60s and later President of the Royal College of Surgeons

'A theatre sister on the fourth floor West thought one of the patients was behaving oddly. When he then climbed out on a window ledge, the sister went out after him. The houseman saw what was happening and went out on the window ledge on the other side of the patient. Both put their lives at risk and were each awarded the George Cross.' **Retired anaesthetist**

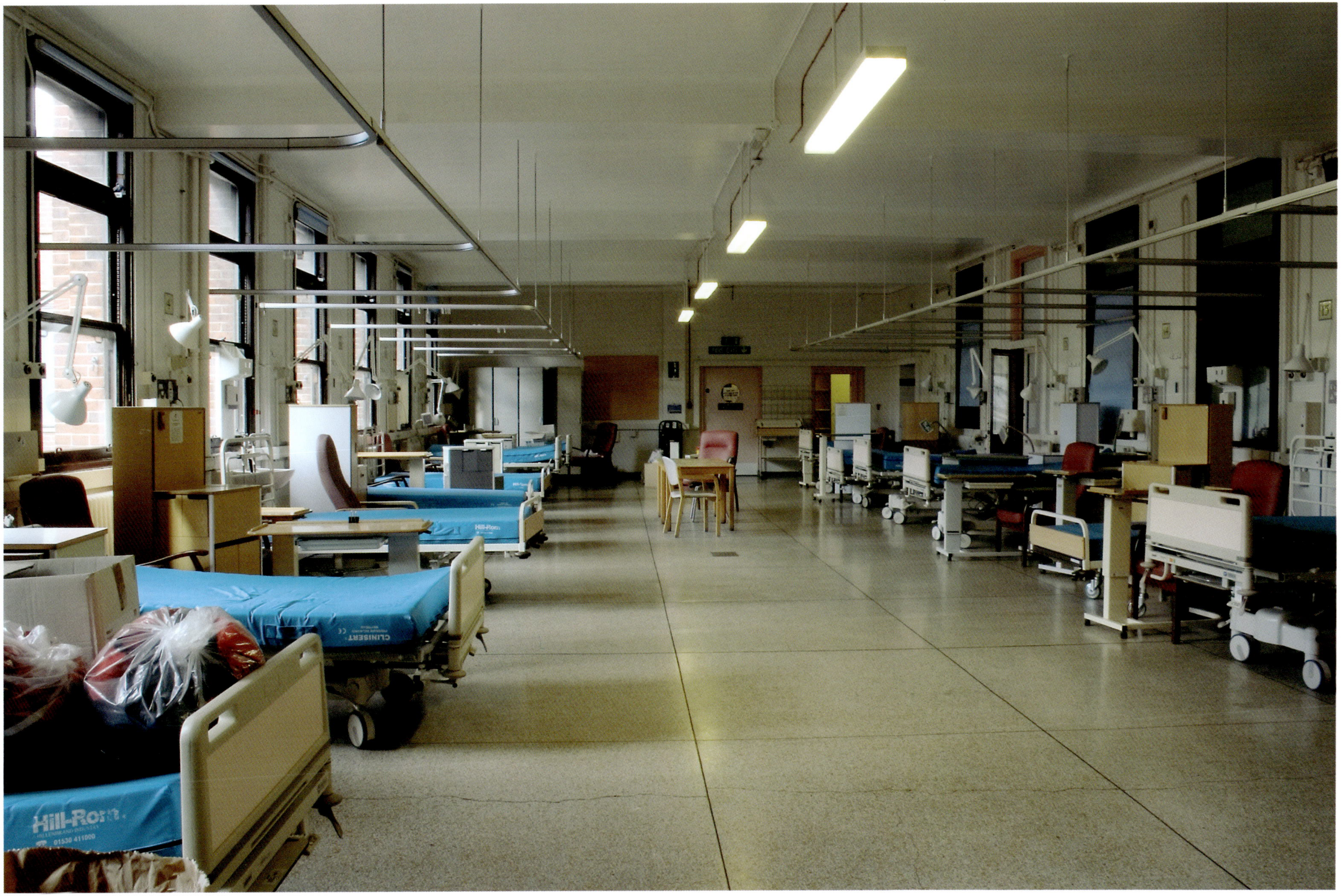
Hill-Rom

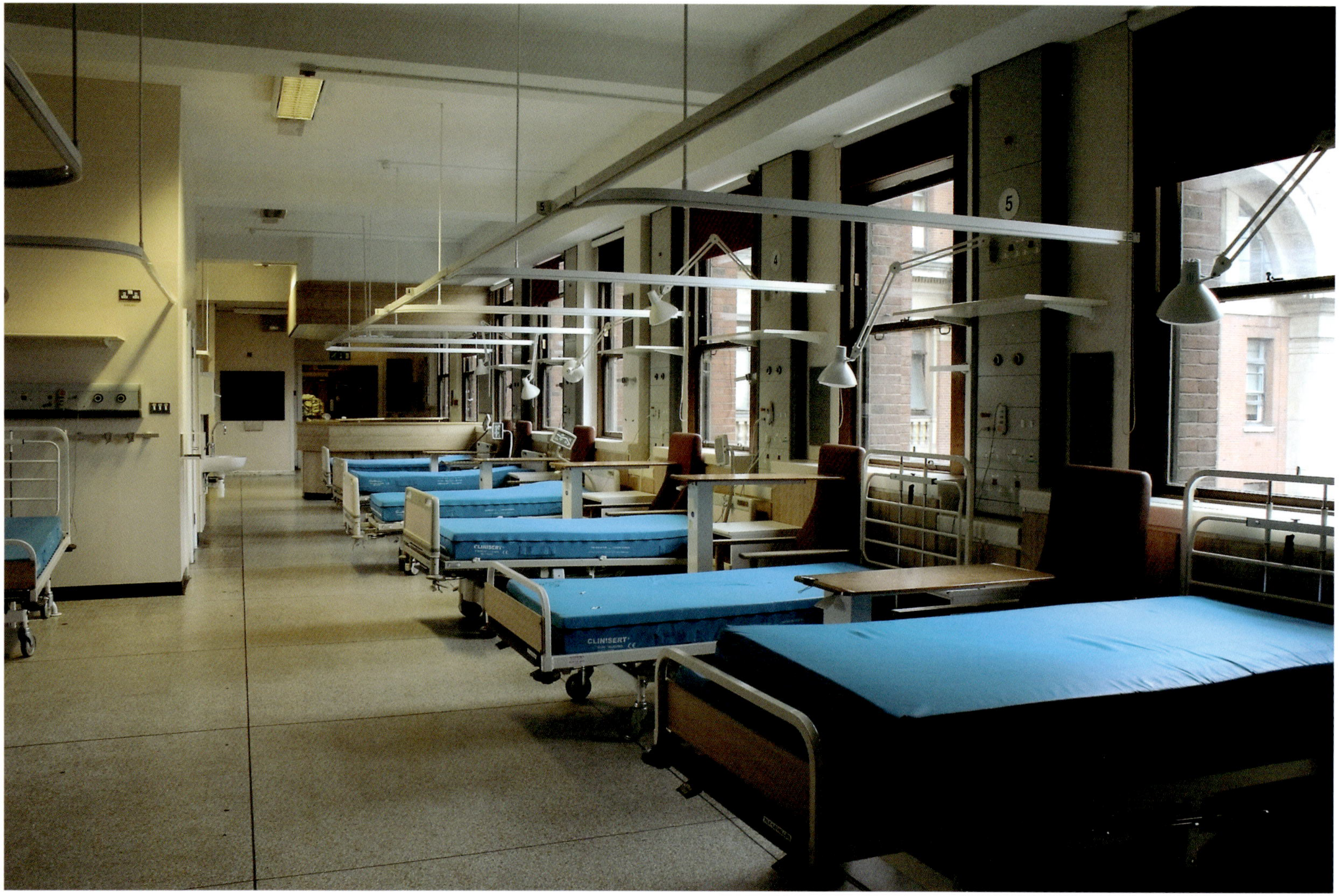
5
CLINISERT

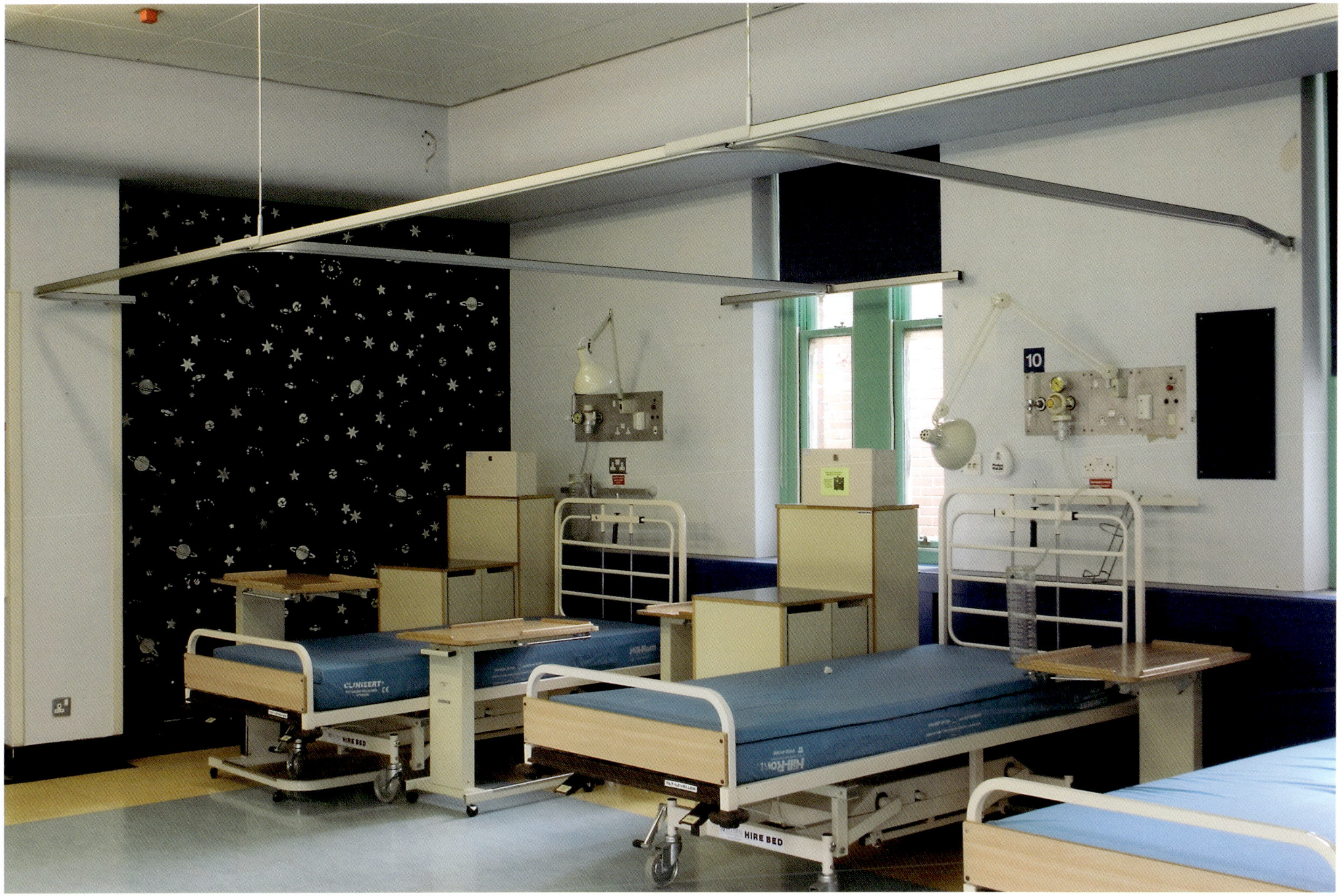
10
HIRE BED
HIRE BED

'In 1982, as a third year psychiatric nursing student at Banstead Hospital, I had a six week placement at The Middlesex. My first impressions were that the nurses were really posh compared to the motley crew we were, all pink shimmer and pearl studs – very Home Counties. They were, however, very friendly and welcoming and did lots of teaching. The ward was really small but we were kept busy all the same.' **Nurse consultant**

'I trained as a nurse at The Middlesex between 1947 and 1952 and worked on all the surgical wards. On night duty we would cook bacon and eggs for starving housemen, many of whom went on to become eminent surgeons.' **Chair of Middlesex Nurses League**

'When Broderip ward was opened as an AIDs ward, this was seen as very portentious and the way forward but in the event, it was later no longer required and was eventually closed.'
Past Bloomsbury Health Authority Chairman

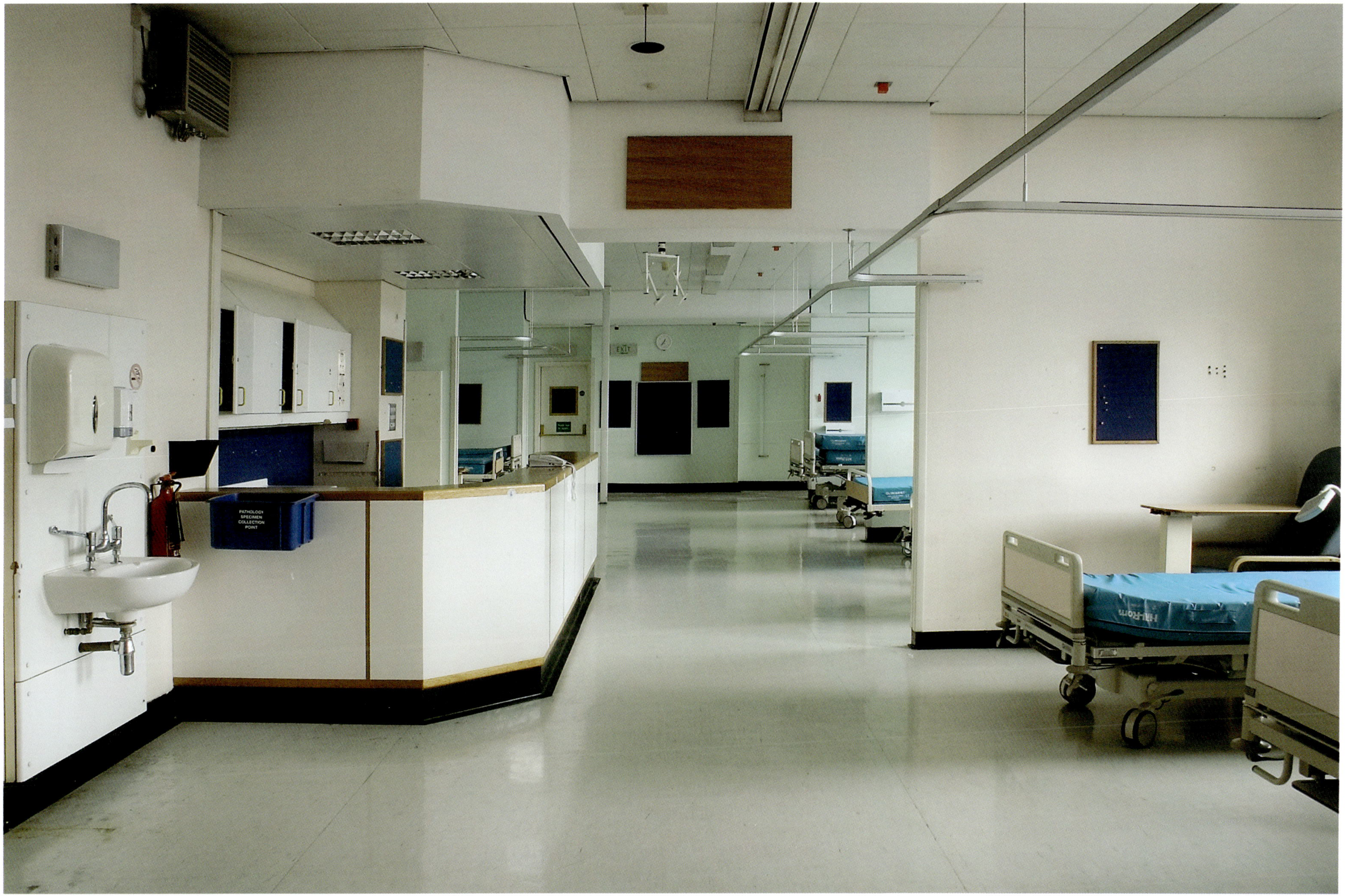
PATHOLOGY
SPECIMEN
COLLECTION
POINT
EXIT

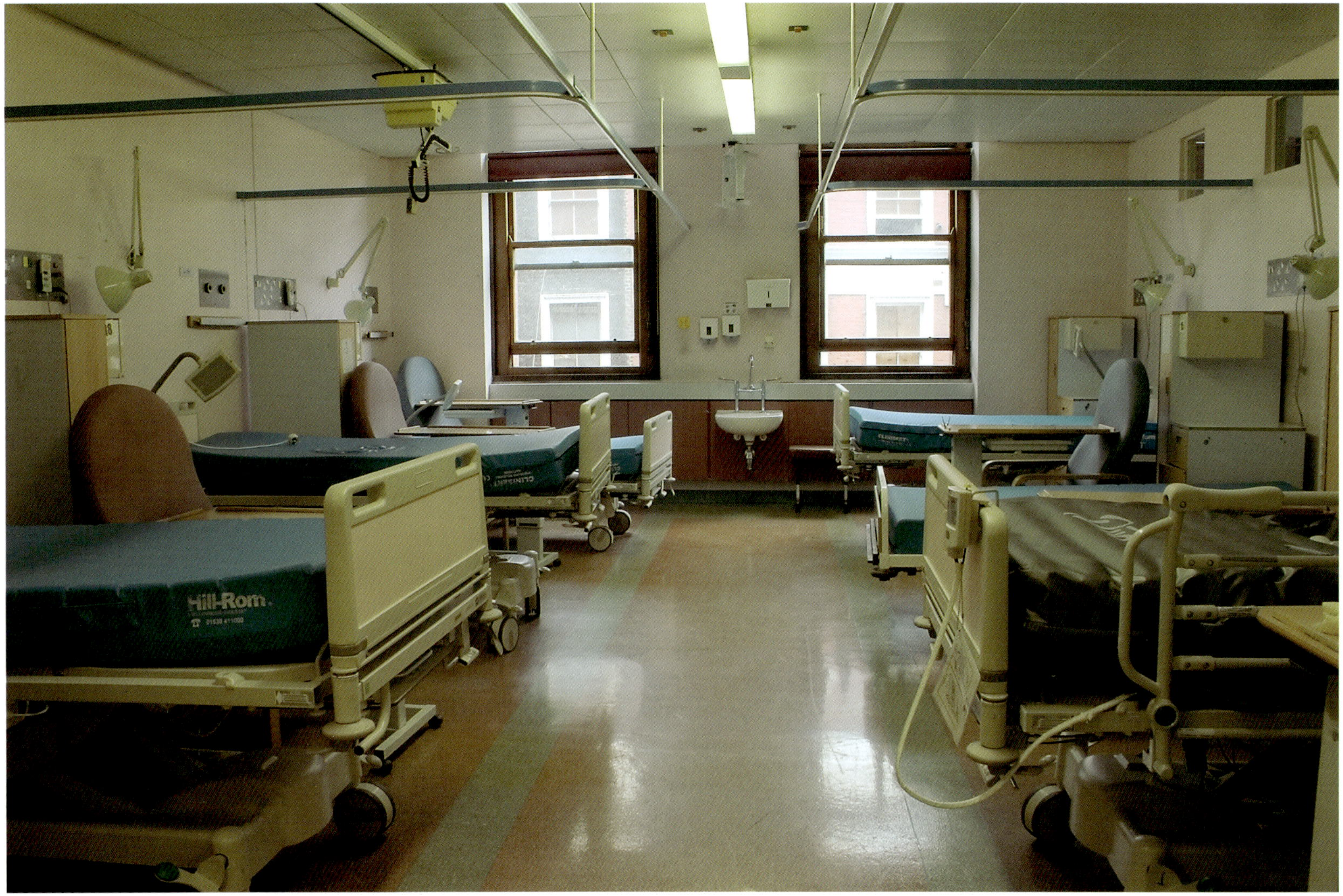
Hill-Rom

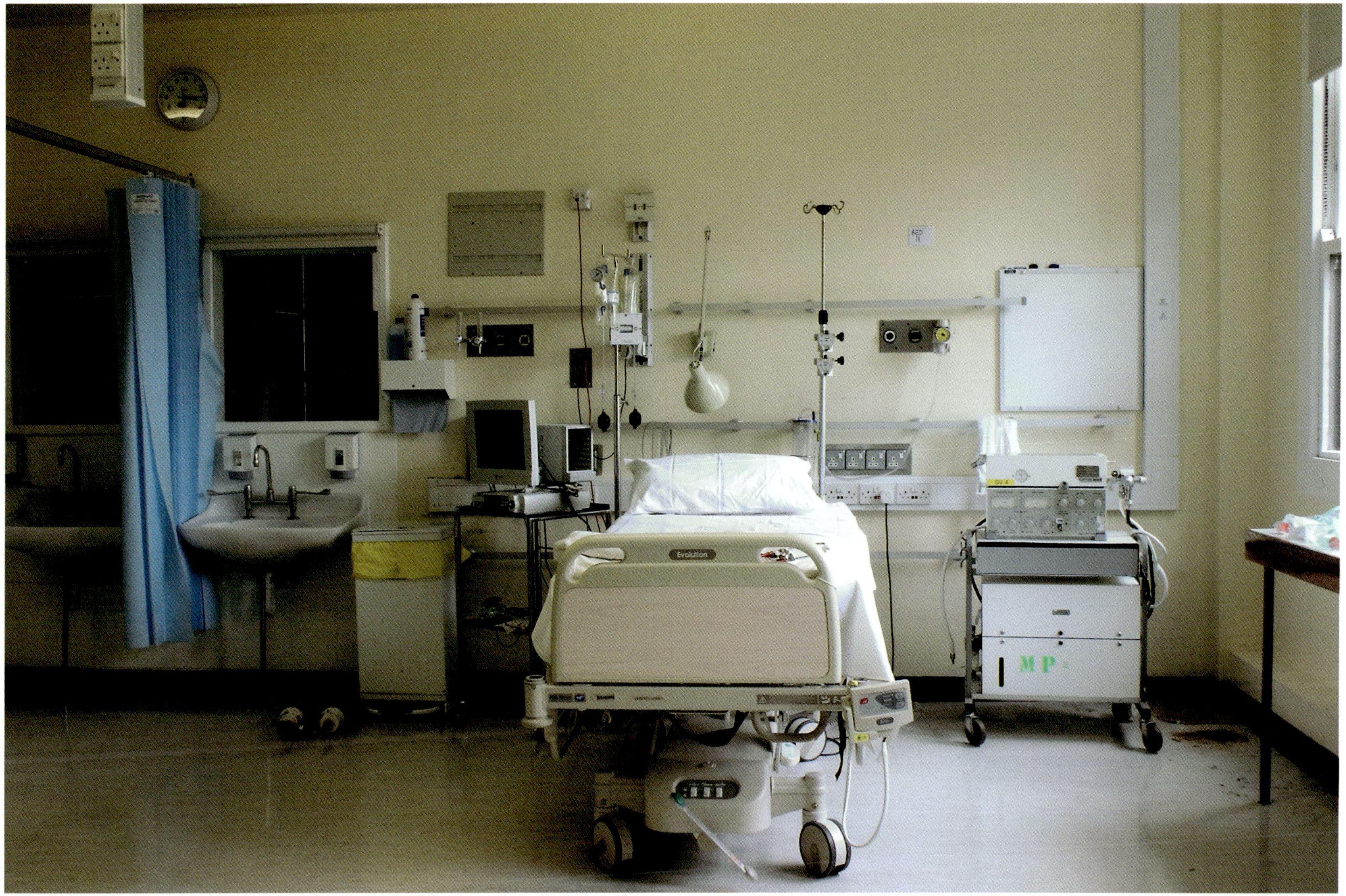
Evolution
MP

'Going round some wards, I remember staff saying how difficult it was to plug in all the equipment needed at the bedside when you only had one round three pin plug. This was just one example of the difference between the quality of medicine at The Middlesex and the quality of the building.' **Past Bloomsbury Health Authority Chairman**

'Medical students used to climb out and run along the ledges outside the wards on the crosspiece as a challenge.'
Medical student in the 60s and later President of the Royal College of Surgeons

'Happy and exhausted after a long labour, I remember looking out of the circular windows on the maternity ward and thinking – well we've done it now, life's never going to be the same – my husband went out and bought champagne and meringues on Goodge Street.' ***Mother, maternity unit in the 70s***

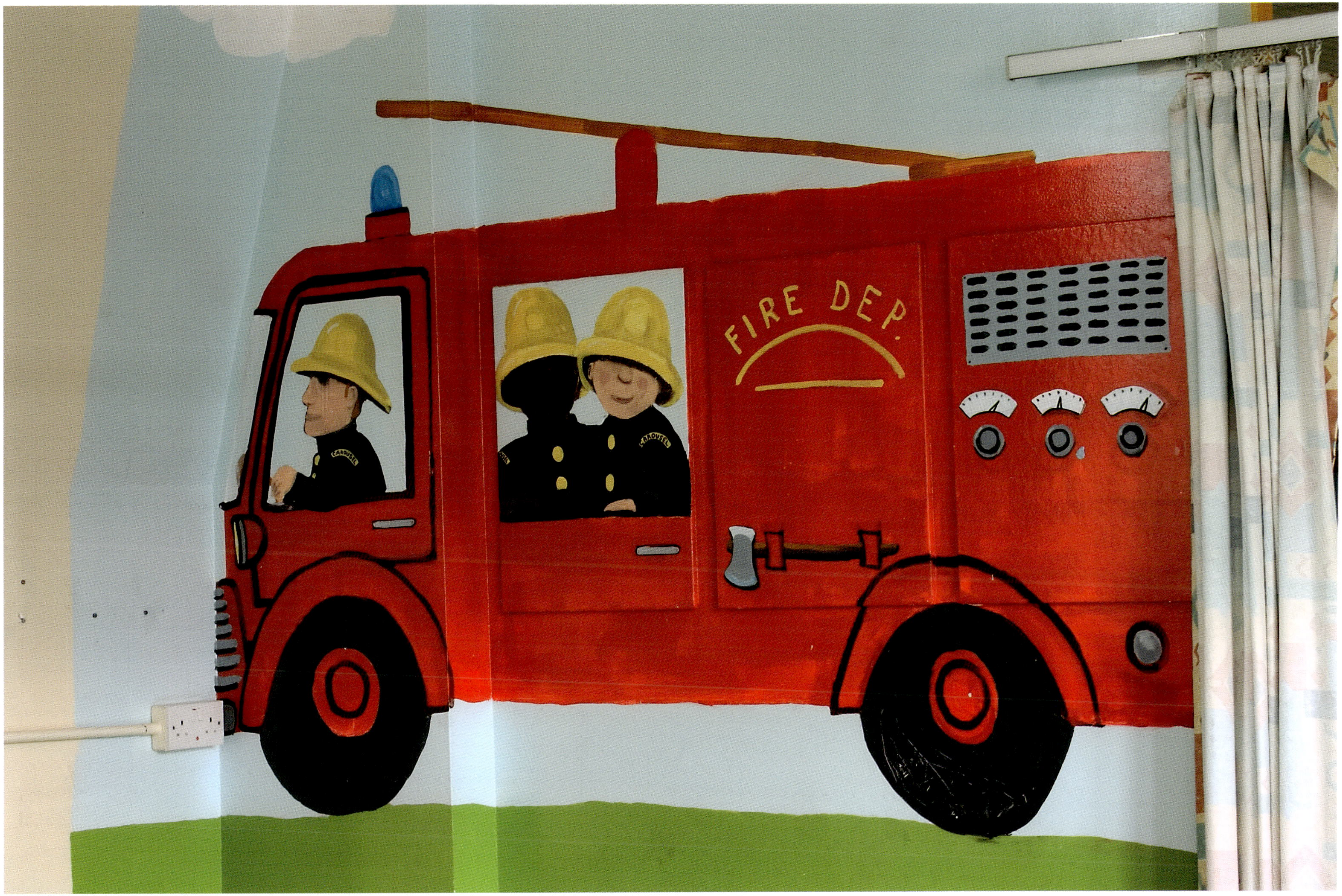
FIRE DEP.

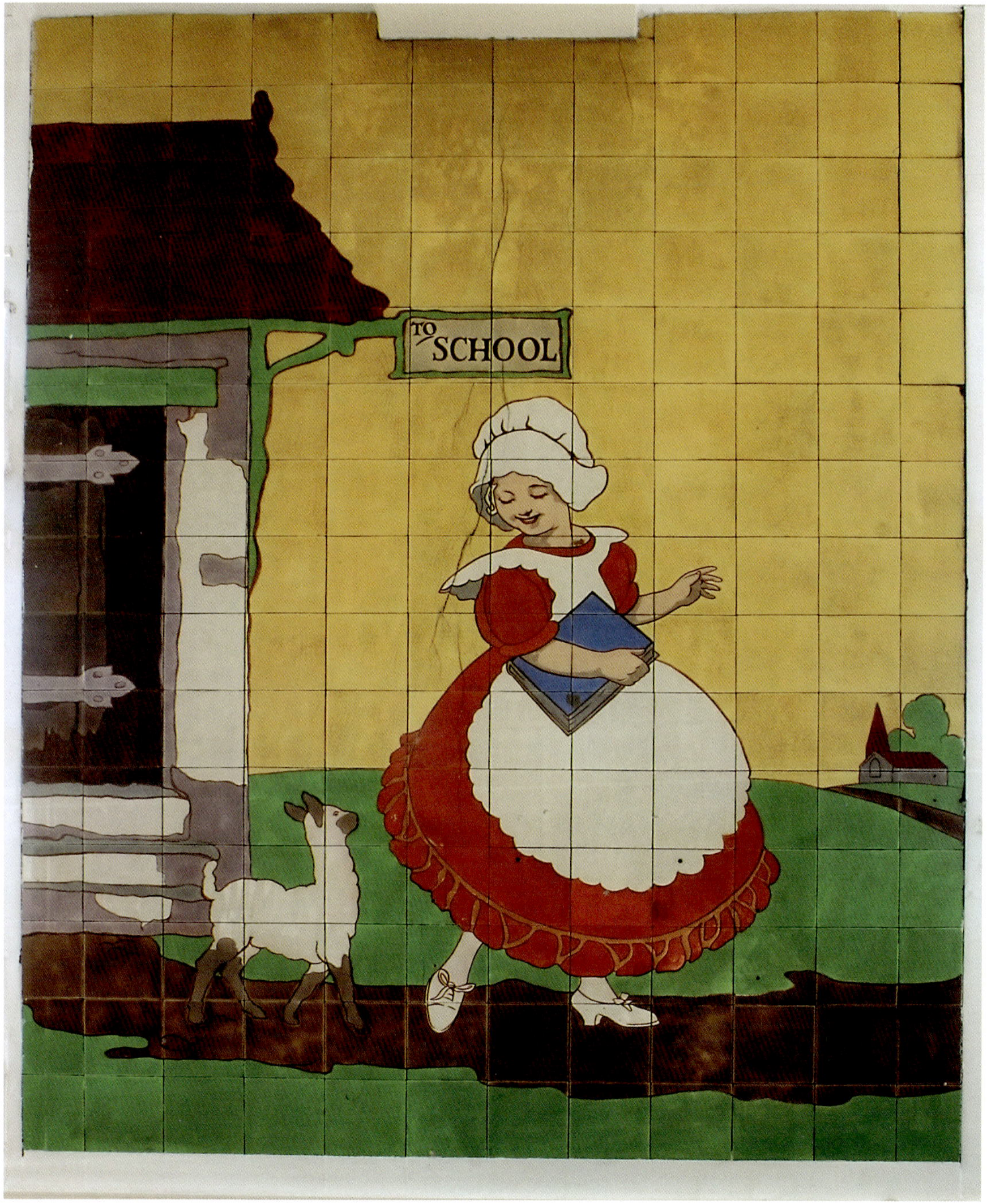
TO SCHOOL

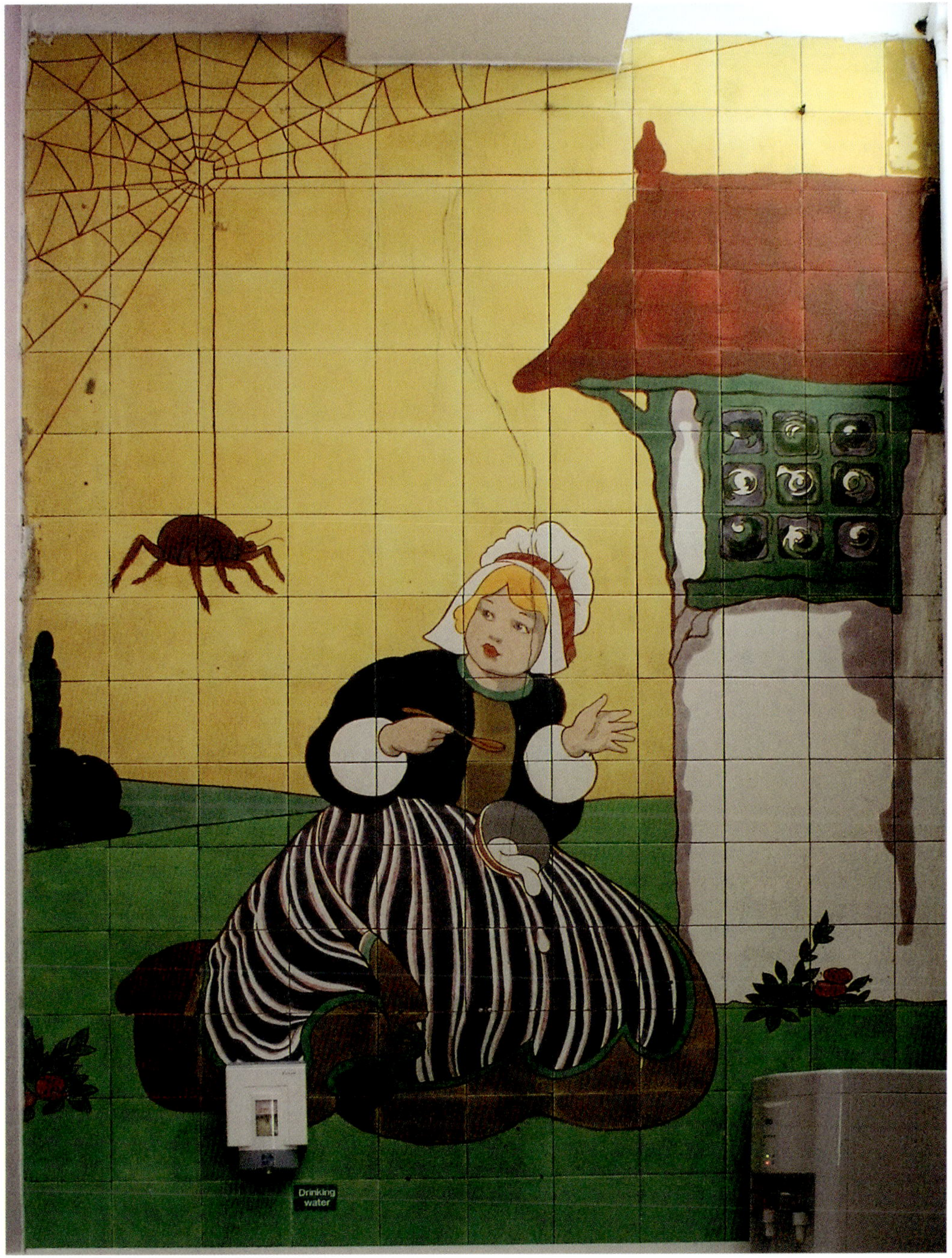
Drinking water

'There was talk in the past of a ghost in the Cancer wing – a grey lady who used to stand by the bedside of patients who were about to die.'

Hilary St George Saunders, author of 'The Middlesex Hospital' published in 1949

'A patient on one of the oncology wards told me that he had seen a kind lady in grey who asked if he was alright, then she vanished. He died shortly afterwards.' ***Senior nursing officer who trained in the late 40s***

'Lord Astor, when he was Chairman, despite being a very shy man, went round to see all the patients – it must have been difficult for him.' ***Senior nursing officer who trained in the late 40s***

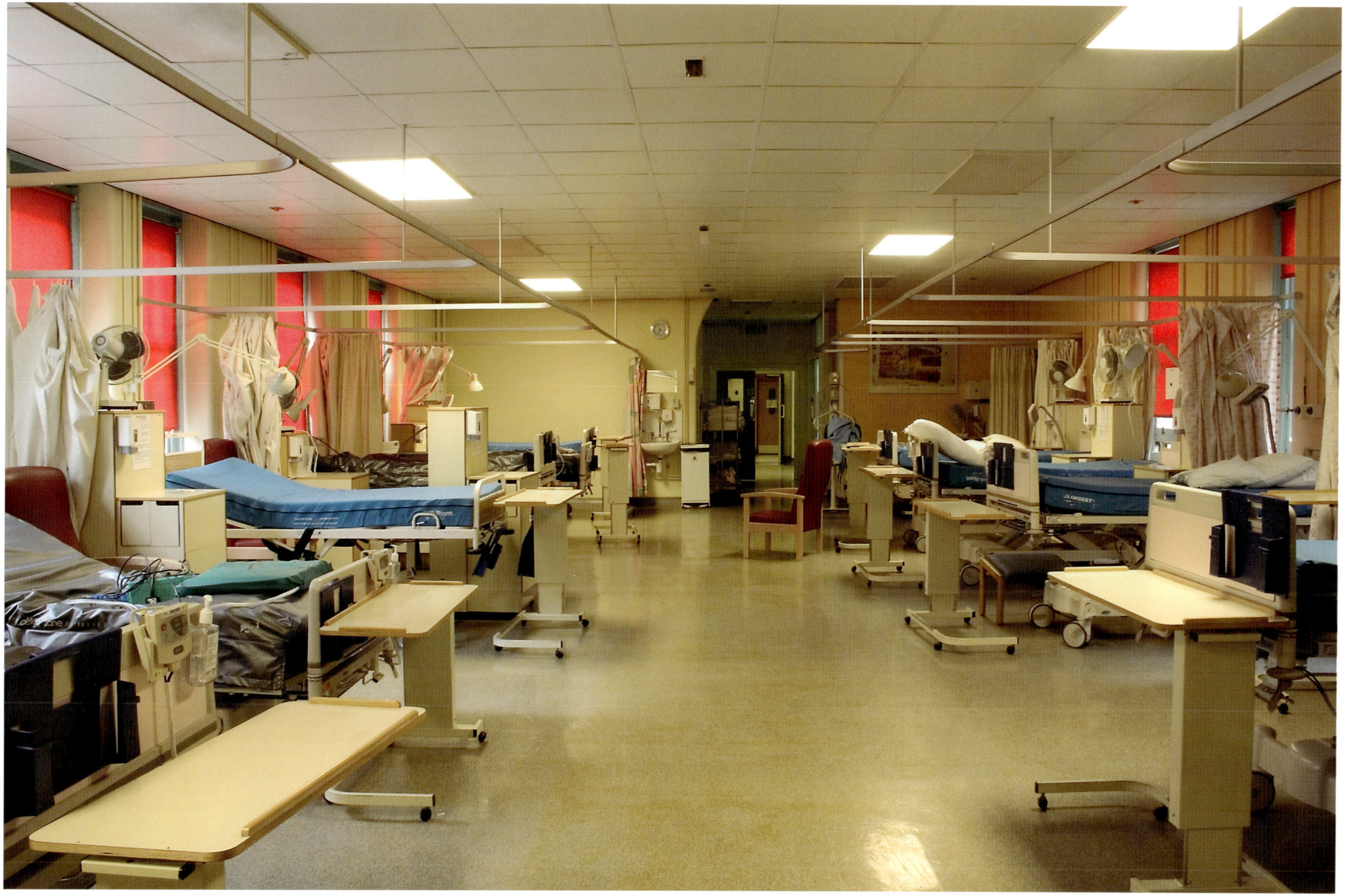

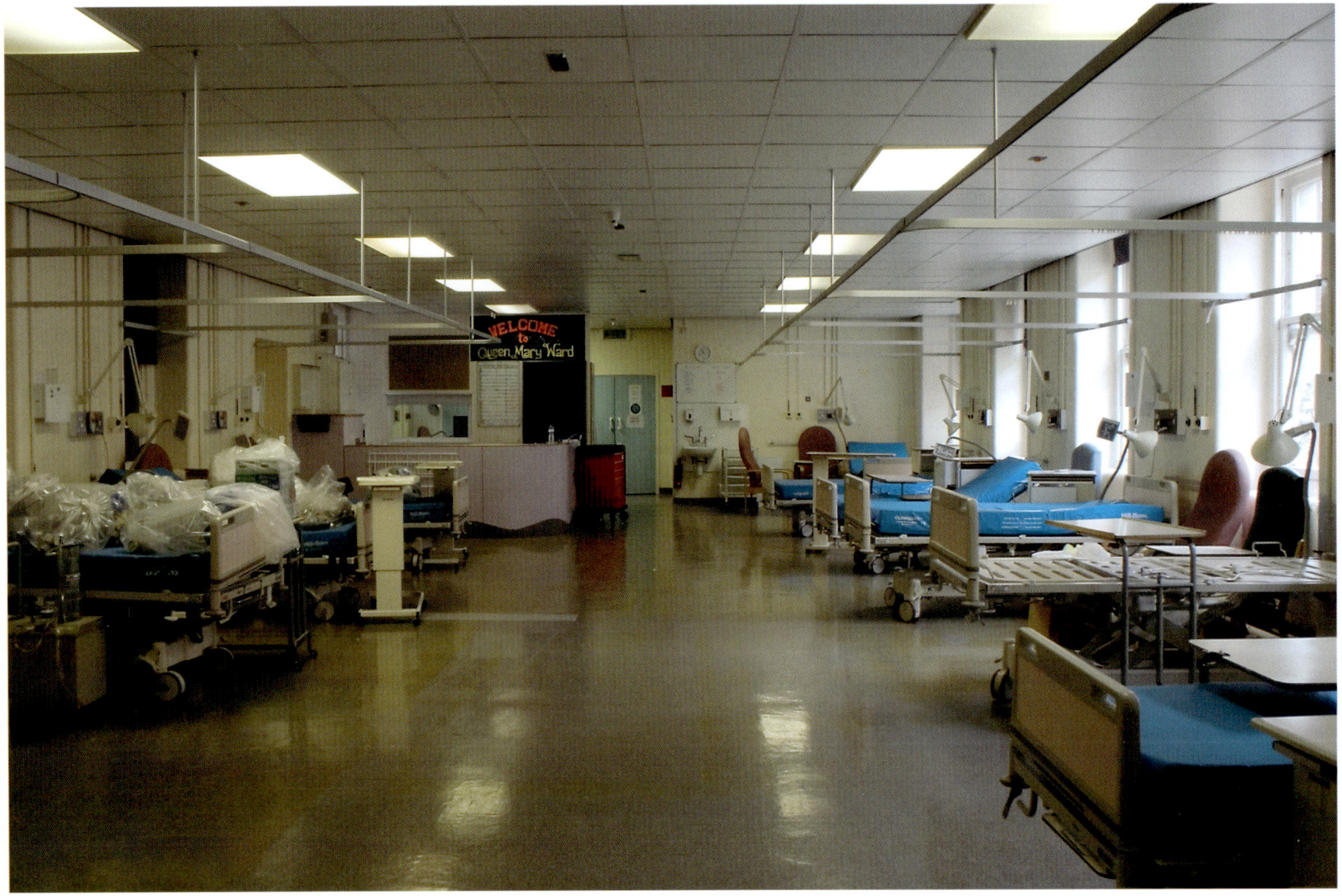
WELCOME
to
Queen Mary Ward

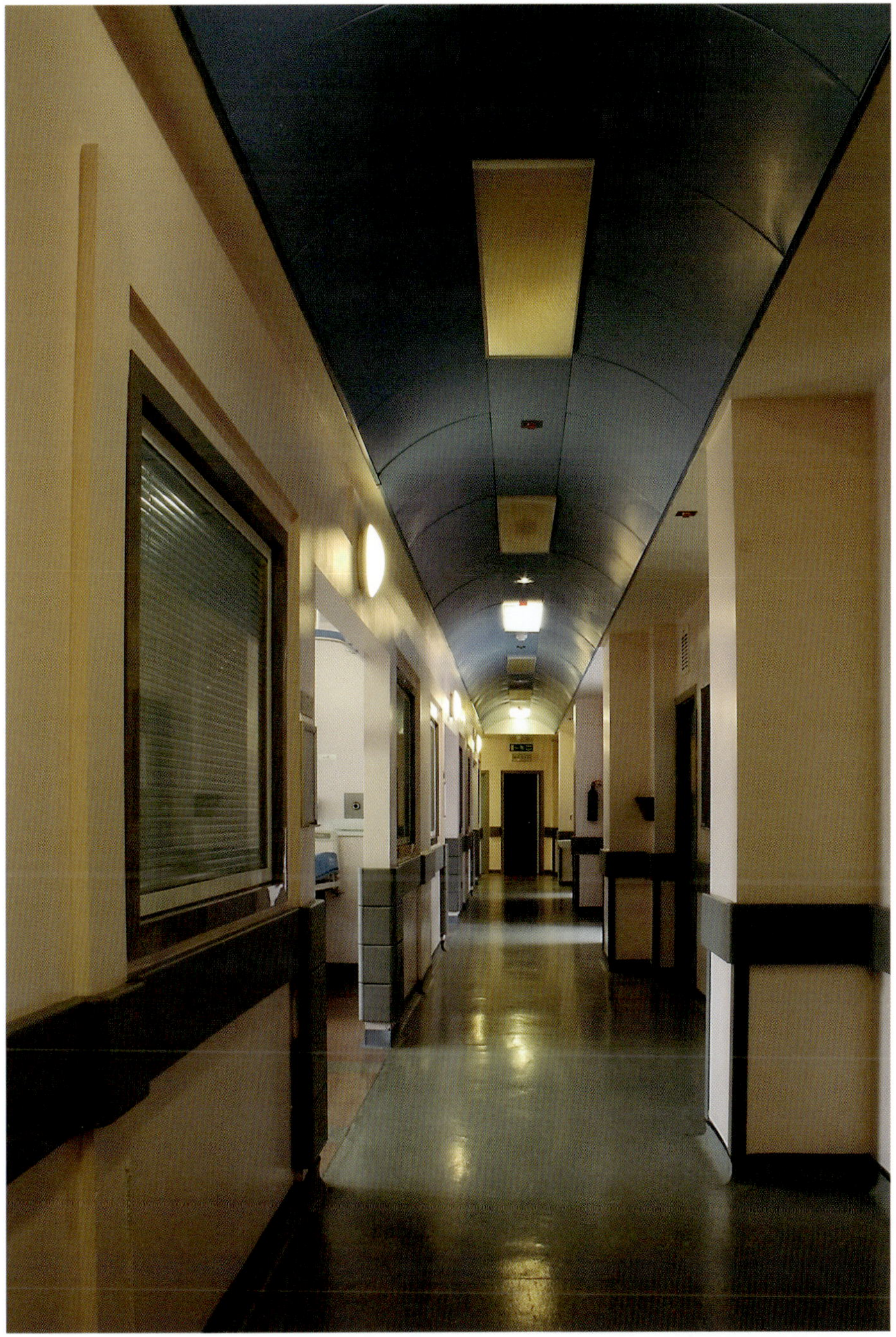

'Being on your own in Bond Street ward at night could sometimes send a tingle down your spine. Once another nurse, who was in the office, came rushing out to find me and see if I was OK. She said I'd tapped her on the shoulder but I hadn't been near the office.' **Senior staff nurse**

'In the early days of cardiac surgery, patients had a high death rate – doctors had a bed on the ward because they had to get up to measure potassium levels every hour.'
Medical student in the 60s and later President of the Royal College of Surgeons

'In those days there was no cardiac resuscitation – you just had adrenal by the bedside. It was difficult to find beds with hard boards to resuscitate patients as most beds had springs.' **Sister who trained in the 50s**

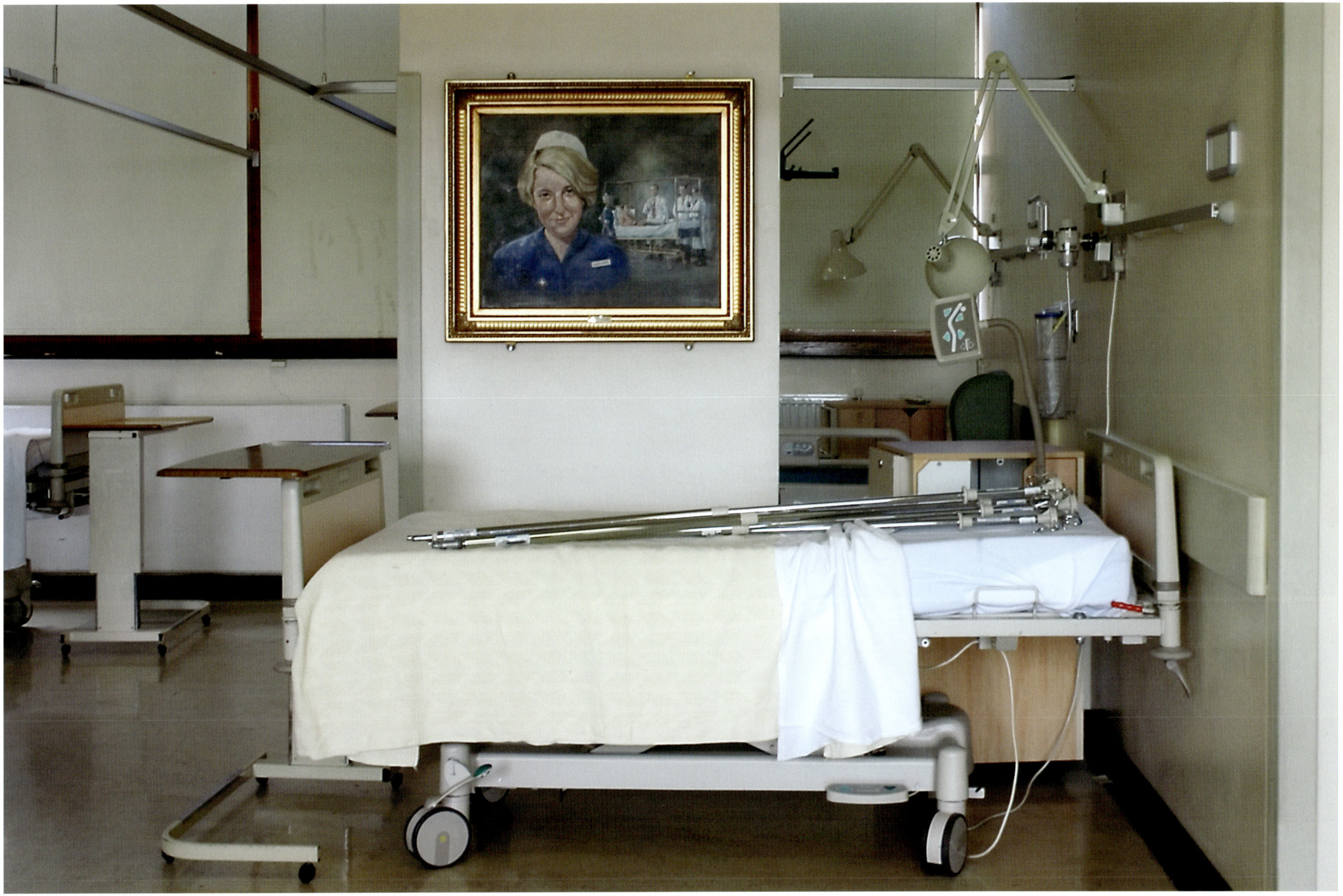

'The glass fronted cupboards in the basement used to hold old leather bound hand written ledgers of patient records and theatre books, many of which went back to the 1800s.' **Retired surgeon**

'In the 1960s, the 200 year old patient archives in the basement provided very valuable historical data for a study of untreated breast cancer patients. This study showed that some of these patients were still alive 20-30 years later.' **Radiotherapy consultant**

'You could easily get lost in the underground corridors if you took a wrong turning. I met my wife, down in those corridors – she heard my booming voice from a distance.'

Medical student in the 60s and later President of the Royal College of Surgeons

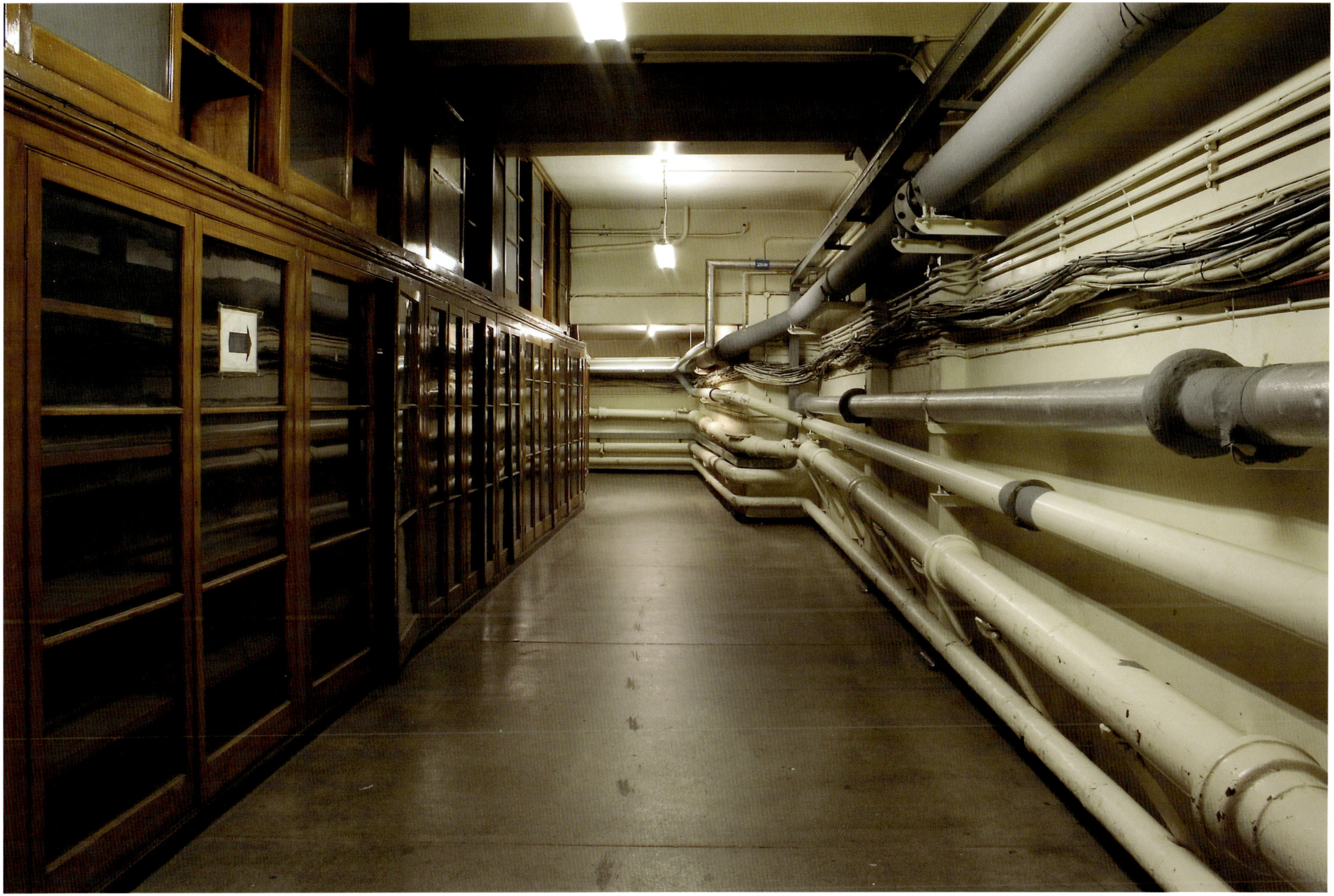

'Nurses really enjoyed the swimming pool in John Astor House – I learned to dive there.' **Nurse**

'The pool in John Astor House was amazing. I'd go and do 20 lengths after waking up after night duty. In those days you did nights for seven days, then had a week off and one weekend a month.' **Sister**

'There used to be an inter-hospital swimming competition which took place in the John Astor House pool.'
Sister who trained in the 50s

'During the shooting season, Lord Astor would send 100 birds up to the Nurses Home and invited sisters down to Hever Castle.' **Retired surgeon**

'Days out for sisters used to be organised at the Astor's residence at Folly Farm designed by Lutyens.'
Nurse consultant ICU

'There used to be a silver service lunch and dinner for sisters in the dining room in John Astor House. Hugh and Emi Lu Astor used to send a coach and invite 25 ward sisters on their day off to their Foley Farm near Newbury, where they had use of all the facilities for the day. Two sisters each year were also invited down to their properties in the South of France for a holiday.' **Retired clinical service manager**

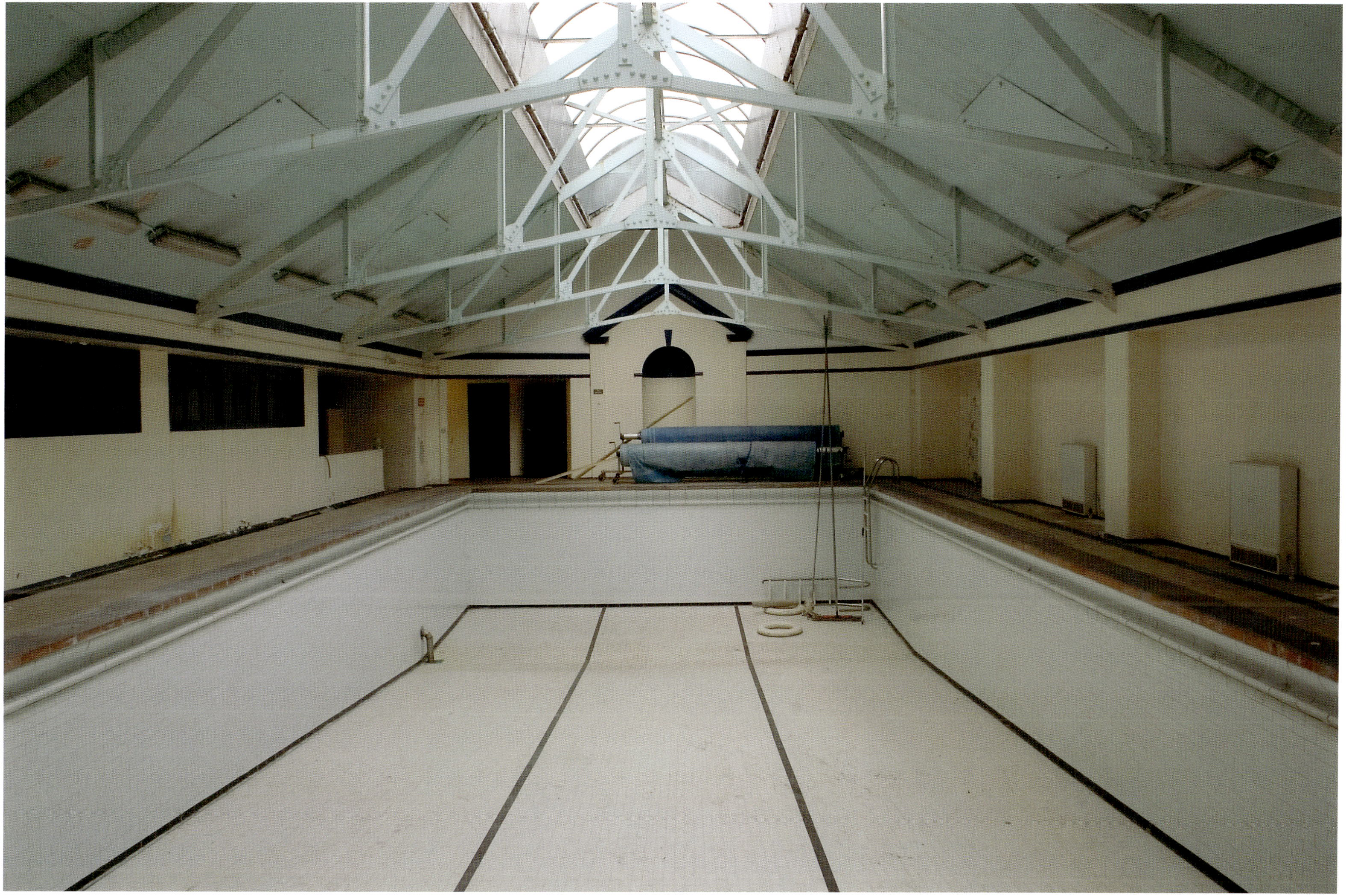

'The courtyard was one of the hospital's great benefits. Many patients found solace there away from all the activity on the wards.' **Retired surgeon**

'The League of Friends took great pride in keeping the courtyard garden in good shape.'
Past President of the League of Friends

'The courtyard was an important space – group surgical department photographs were taken out on the patio and hockey and rugby club photographs in the garden.'
Medical student in the 60s and later President of the Royal College of Surgeons

'The matron's office used to be in what became the physio gym – it was wood panelled and had a view overlooking the courtyard garden.' **Retired clinical service manager**

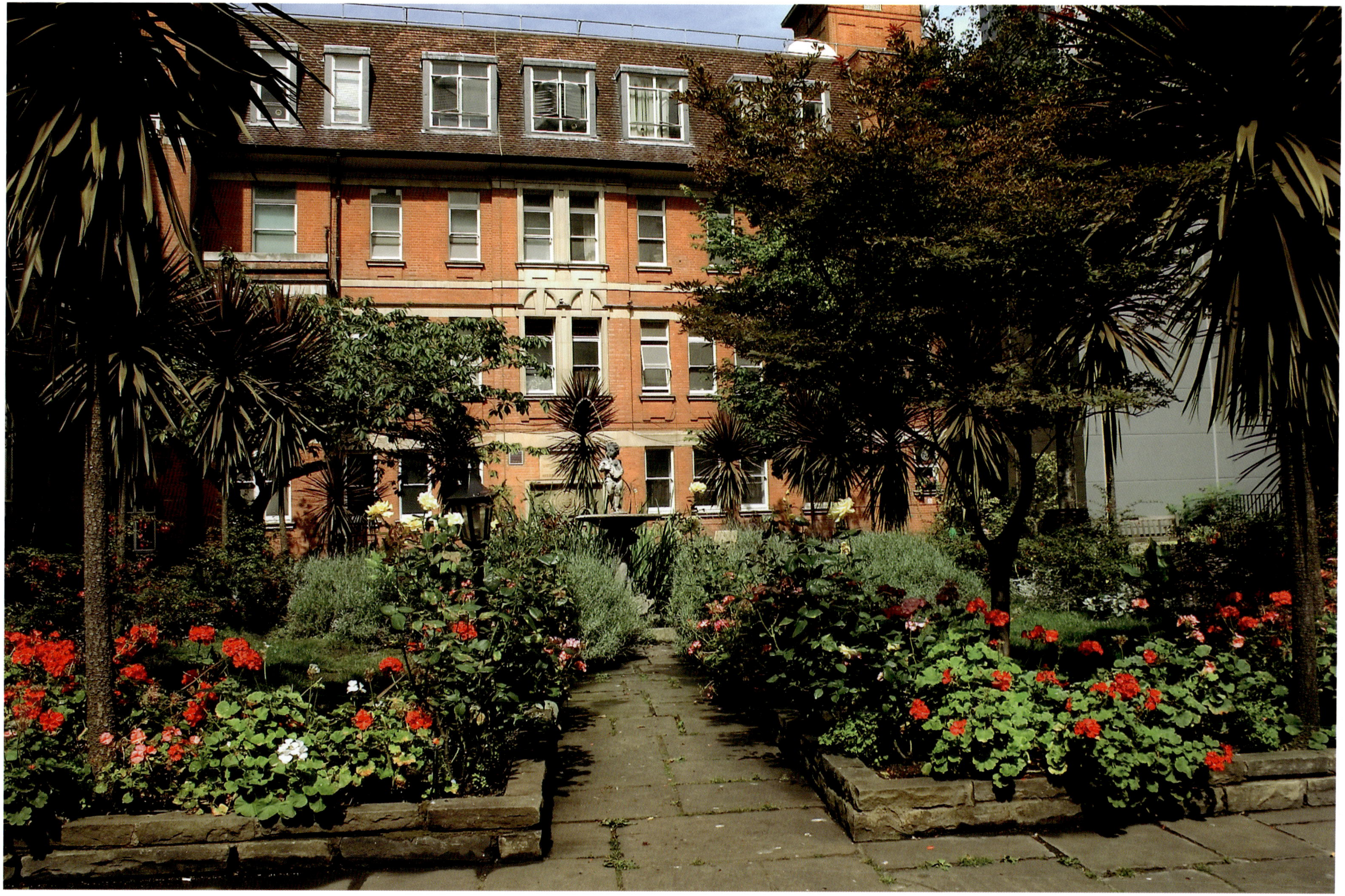

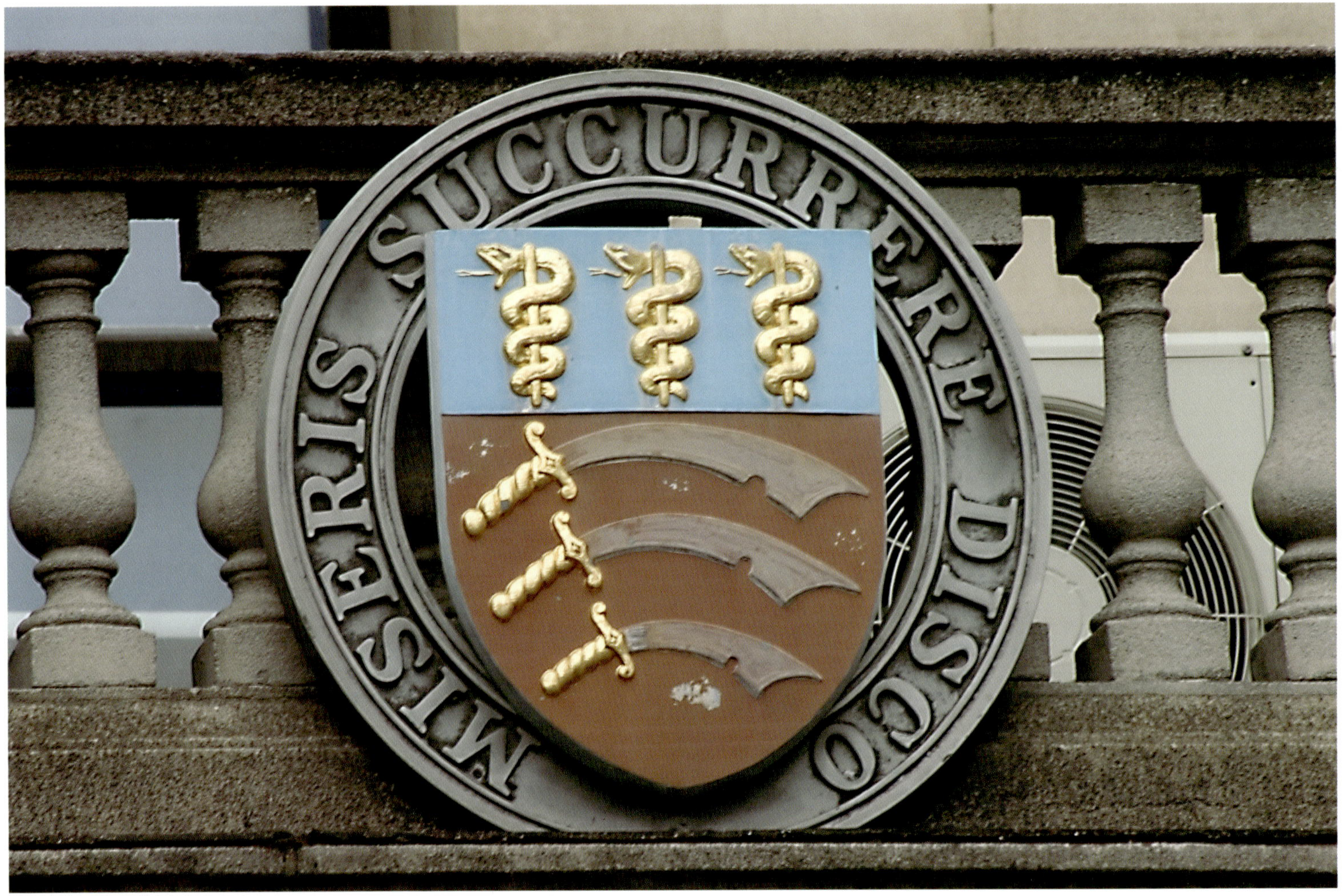
MISERIS SUCCURRERE DISCO

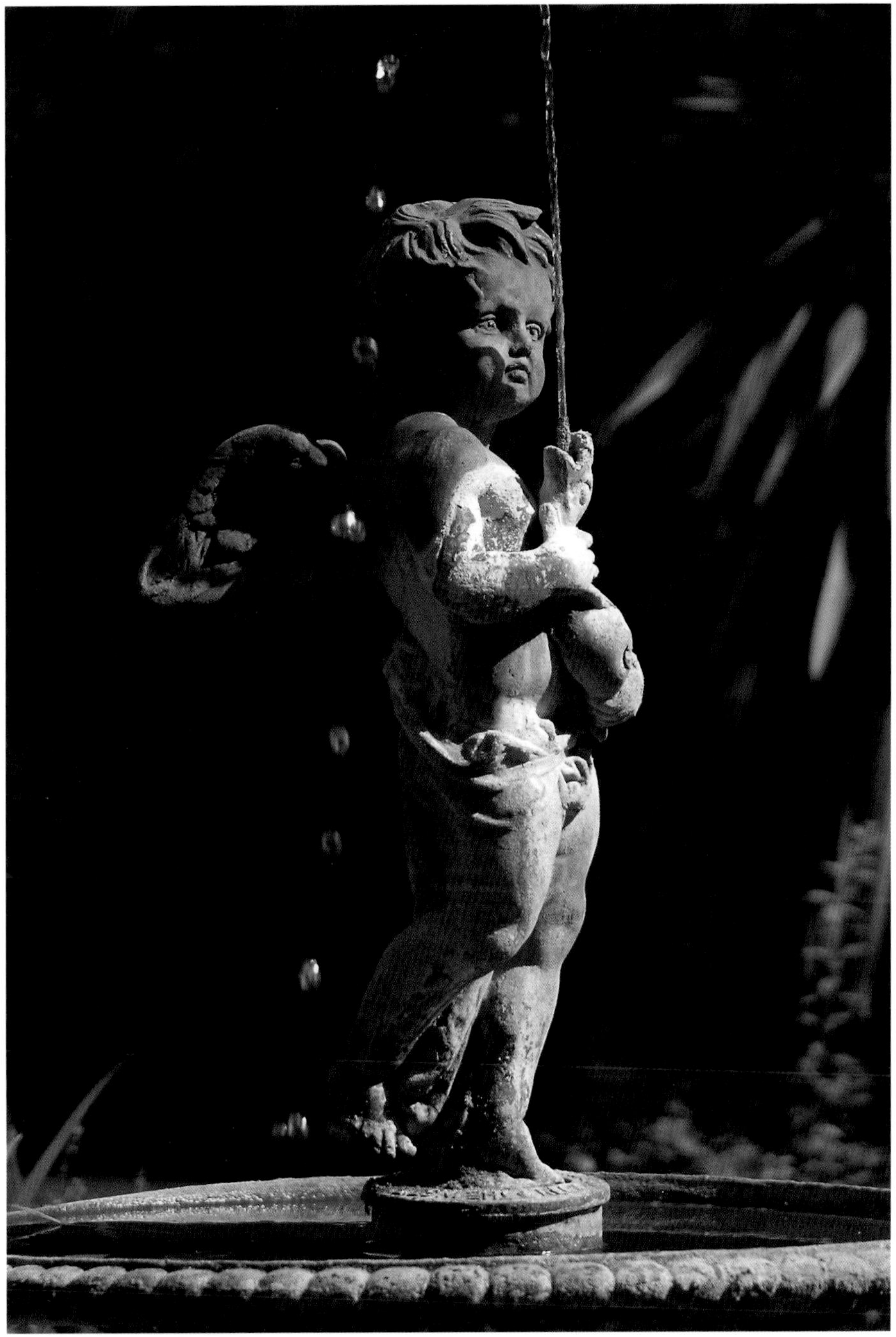

List of Photographs